PREVENTION'S

Quick & Healthy

FAMILY FAVORITES

COOKBOOK

PREVENTION'S
Quick & Healthy
FAMILY FAVORITES
COOKBOOK

225 Delicious Recipes

from the Food Editors

of *Prevention* Health Books®

RODALE

In all Rodale cookbooks, our mission is to provide delicious and nutritious recipes. Our recipes also meet the standards of the Rodale Test Kitchen for dependability, ease, practicality, and, most of all, great taste. To give us your comments, call (800) 848-4735.

The recipes in this book have been previously published by Rodale Inc. in *Prevention's Quick and Healthy Low-Fat Cooking* series

© 2000 by Rodale Inc.

Printed in the United States of America on acid-free , recycled paper ♻

Cover and Interior Designer: Tanja Lipinski Cole

Library of Congress Cataloging-in-Publication Data

Prevention's quick and healthy family favorites cookbook : 225 delicious recipes / from the food editors of Prevention Health Books.
p.   cm.
"The recipes in this book have been previously published by Rodale Inc. in Prevention's quick and healthy low-fat cooking series"—Colophon.
Includes index.
ISBN 1–57954–310–3 hardcover
1. Low-fat diet—Recipes.   I. Prevention Magazine Health Books.   II. Prevention's quick and healthy low-fat cooking.
RM237.7 .P739   2000
641.5'638—dc21   00–036915

2   4   6   8   10   9   7   5   3   1   hardcover

Visit us on the Web at www.rodalecookbooks.com, or call us toll-free at (800) 848-4735.

WE **INSPIRE** AND **ENABLE** PEOPLE TO IMPROVE
THEIR LIVES AND THE WORLD AROUND THEM

contents

Healthy Habits— Now and Forever

THE FAT-FIGHTING EDGE

America is the land of plenty—plenty of burgers, plenty of pizza, plenty of apple pie. The result for too many of us is extra pounds that sap our energy and threaten our health. Clearly, the excess weight has to go, but getting rid of it is never easy. Even when you are successful, those unwanted pounds have a way of picking up your scent like a pack of bloodhounds hot on your trail. Before you know it, they've once again got you surrounded.

So how do you lose those dogs—er, pounds—once and for all? You have to change your scent. Become a new person. Become a person who no longer leads an overweight lifestyle with its overweight habits. And the trick is to do it without taxing your willpower, without subjecting yourself to undue deprivation and without adding rules and regulations that you can't wait to be rid of.

In other words, you have to create a new lifestyle that you can follow long

enough to have it become second nature. You want a friend that hangs around for the rest of your life, guarding you against ever gaining weight again.

Understand the Basics

Does the phrase "look before you leap" ring a bell? You can't make an honest commitment to do something unless you have some idea of what is required. So let's go through the healthy-lifestyle facts of life.

The first fact of life is that you can't lose 30 pounds in a month. Nor would you want to. After all, the goal isn't just to lose weight; it's to keep the pounds off permanently. And most experts agree that you have the best chances of doing that if you take a gradual approach—dropping no more than one pound a week.

The second fact of life is that in order to lose that pound a week, you need to establish a daily deficit of 500 calories. That requires some combination of the right foods and the right exercise. Most weight-loss experts favor a program in which you cut 200 calories of fat (roughly 22 grams of fat) from your daily diet and burn off 300 calories through exercise to achieve the magic number. (When it comes to diet, it's actually better to count grams of fat instead of calories.)

The third fact of life is that the first two facts are useless unless you follow them consistently and maintain them long after excess pounds are gone. That means being comfortable with the changes you make and not demanding more of yourself than you are prepared to give.

Fat Facts

The average American's diet is approximately 40 percent fat. And because fat calories are more readily converted into body fat, those kinds of calories are the first ones you want to reduce. But the question is, by how much?

Diet experts advocate a fat intake of no more than 25 percent of total calories. What does that really mean? Well, for a woman to maintain a weight of 130 pounds, for instance, she should take in about 1,600 calories a day. If only 25 percent of those calories come from fat, that's 400 calories' worth. Since each gram of fat is good for 9 calories, that's an upper level of 44 grams of fat a day. If you are a 160-pound woman eating 2,000 calories a day (at the 40 percent fat level), you're currently consuming about 89 grams of fat. To reach a streamlined 130 pounds, you need to figure out how to be satisfied with 45 fewer grams of fat per day. But not all at once.

As we mentioned before, to jump onto the pound-a-week weight-loss wagon, you need to cut 500 calories a day: 200 from your daily intake and 300 through exercise. With exercise making its hefty contribution, all that is really required to get the weight-loss wagon rolling is that you bid farewell to approximately 22 grams of fat per day.

After a certain amount of time, your 22-gram fat deficit, along with exercise, can slim your body to a point where it functions so efficiently that you stop losing weight. At this point, having become used to the dietary changes you've made, you can then go ahead and cut your fat intake far enough to reach a fat budget that corresponds to your dream maintenance weight.

While sheer instinct may tell you to grit your teeth and cut all the fat in sight, hoping your willpower holds out, that is the last thing you should do. "Completely eliminating your problem foods may set you up for failure," says Judith S. Stern, Sc.D., professor of nutrition and internal medicine at the University of California, Davis. "You have to determine what those foods are and find ways to replace them if you can't control your appetite for them."

Diane Hanson, Ph.D., a lifestyle specialist at the Pritikin Longevity Center in Santa Monica, California, thinks of it as leveraging your food choices: "Doable changes that make a big difference. For example, if two or three tablespoons of blue-cheese dressing at lunch are dumping 16 or 24 grams of fat onto your daily intake, a small packet of low-fat dressing brought from home can shave off the grams and still leave you satisfied."

The concept of food substitutes is nothing new. But what makes them so exciting now is the ever-growing selection of low-fat products that are on the market. The difference between a regular meat lasagna entrée and a low-fat one translates into a fat savings of 7 grams. A nonfat, fruit-filled breakfast pastry can save you 16 grams of fat if you substitute it for the "real thing." Suddenly, dropping your fat intake for life doesn't look like such hungry work. But whatever you drop should be dropped for good. So choose carefully, or the pounds will return.

Before you lull yourself to sleep with visions of breakfast-pastry weight loss, remember this: At some point, you're going to have to sweat. A study conducted by Dr. Susan Kayman, Dr. William Bruvold and Dr. Judith Stern at the University of California found that 90 percent of the participants who kept the weight off exercised regularly.

The Exercise Equation

"To my mind, exercise has been undervalued with respect to weight loss," says Dr. Hanson. "As a matter of fact, when you look at what determines the continuation of a healthy lifestyle, exercise turns out to be the biggest behavioral driver."

It helps you look good and feel even better. It gives you a sense of accomplishment and mastery over your situation. "Research is even showing that exercise may enhance your preference for fruits and vegetables," says Dr. Hanson.

Even if you already like veggies, exercise serves another important purpose. When you lower your calorie intake, your body, with an instinct for survival, slows down its metabolic rate and conserves energy. Exercise turns up the furnace so you become more efficient at burning fat. And to drop a pound a week, you want that furnace stoked to the tune of 300 calories burned a day.

How you accomplish that goal is a matter of what you like to do. But the good news is that even a brisk 45-minute walk will do the trick. But the real trick is to do it every day.

Make the Commitment

The difference between losing weight and losing weight for good is commitment: a truly motivated desire not only to change but also to maintain that change. You can think of your commitment as a lifetime contract with yourself. Of course, we've all cheated on some of our vows to become better, more effective or slimmer. In most cases, the problem isn't our willpower but our initial commitment. It just wasn't strong enough.

Before starting your new, lighter life, you need to make sure that you're revved and ready to do it and that the contract you make with yourself is so strong that the Supreme Court—or a tempting éclair with your name on it—couldn't break it. Here's how to really, pardon the expression, commit yourself.

Choose the right moment. "It's not easy to begin a program during complicated periods in your life," says Kelly D. Brownell, Ph.D., professor of psychology at Yale University. "Divorce, an illness in the family, problems at work—those are all things that can sap your energy and make your environment less supportive for the changes you want to make."

Of course, some people thrive on complications. A divorce, for example, may be just the motivating kick one person needs to make big changes as part of a whole new lifestyle. "The thing you need to consider," says Dr. Brownell, "is how you respond to complications. If stress, worry and a frantic pace erode your eating plan, making serious lifestyle changes in the midst of what's currently happening may be a mistake."

And you don't want to look just at the present. If you're due for "stormy weather" in the upcoming weeks and months, you may want to bide your time and embark on your new lifestyle once things calm down and the sun comes out again.

Choose the right commitment. Do you want to lose a certain number of pounds, or do you want to lose the bad habits that made you overweight to begin with? While those two goals may seem to be heads and tails of the same coin, the side that lands up after the toss can make all the difference between pounds gone forever and pounds gone for an all-too-brief amount of time.

"If you find yourself fantasizing about the moment when you've lost the weight and your diet is over, you're going to have problems," says Dr. Brownell. "At the point when you've finally reached that all-important number on the scale, there's a chance that your motivation to continue your healthy lifestyle may decrease, leaving you right back where you started."

So to make the commitment that will keep those pounds away forever, focus on the changes you plan to make. "Change your view of success," suggests Dr. Hanson. "Rather than making weight loss your goal, make life-long health your goal. Rather than getting up each morning and heading for the scale, wake up and notice how much better you feel."

"I also find it helpful to think of overweight as a chronic condition," adds Dr. Brownell. "Just as diabetes requires constant maintenance lest it get serious, maintaining your ideal weight requires a lifetime of healthy eating and exercising practices."

Choose the right reason. "Some people lose weight because their husbands or wives want them to," says Jerome Brandon, Ph.D., an exercise physiologist from Georgia State University in Atlanta and member of the American College of Sports Medicine. "The problem is that they make the effort to lose weight for someone else rather than because they themselves are personally motivated to do it. And eventually, they will get tired of doing it."

So do it for yourself and not for someone else.

Get Prepared

Every great journey begins with a great deal of preparation. How far would Christopher Columbus have gotten if he'd just awakened one morning, kissed his wife and headed out to discover the New World without the proper clothes, food, transportation or navigational equipment?

Changing your life is not much different from making a journey. In both cases, the most disappointing thing that can happen is that you have to give up because of difficulties you weren't prepared for. So no matter how charged up you are to start your new life, take some time to make the following preparations.

Educate yourself. If you're going to make lifestyle changes that you expect to practice for the rest of your life, you'd darn well better believe in them. And the best way to believe in something is to know beyond a shadow of a doubt how it works and, more important, why it works.

"First, when it comes to weight loss, there are scientific reasons for why it's best to eat and exercise a certain way," says Dr. Hanson. "If you understand how your body is designed to work, you'll believe in what you're doing and not be so inclined to give it up when the results are not happening as quickly as you want."

Second, by not understanding their body's own weight-loss mechanisms, people often select popular methods that doom them to failure. Then they blame themselves—when they never really had a chance. "You may think that the more calories you deprive yourself of, the faster you'll lose weight, and that's initially true. But if you don't realize that the body slows down its fat-burning furnace when calories are suddenly reduced, you're ultimately in for a big disappointment," says Dr. Hanson. "The only thing that will happen over time is that you'll be hungrier, less inclined to continue your program and still not sure why you aren't maintaining the initial weight loss."

So start out right by getting the facts. Know without a doubt that what you are doing is right and will eventually provide you with the results you want regardless of how things appear to be going on a day-to-day basis.

Find substitutes for eating. "When talking to patients, I often ask them why they overeat, why are they doing something that they know is ultimately harmful," says Dean Ornish, M.D., director of the Preventive Medicine Research Institute in Sausalito, California, and author of the best-selling *Eat More, Weigh Less.* "And the answer often is that it helps to get them through the day. They may feel alienated or isolated, and eating helps them deal with the pain. One patient described how food temporarily fills the void and numbs the pain."

According to Dr. Ornish, change is not brought about solely by focusing on new behaviors such as changing your eating habits and exercising. You need to address the underlying reasons for your behaviors. Otherwise, the problem remains and will eventually sabotage all your good intentions and commitments.

If some form of mental stress is behind your eating problem, you'll need to find a nonfattening substitute. Relaxation techniques and spending more time with friends are both great alternatives that are far lower in calories than a banana split.

Remove roadblocks. Visualize the changes you want to make, then visualize all the things that could keep you from doing them. "It could be that you are unwilling to start exercising," says Dr. Brownell. "But if you dig a little deeper, you may find that the reason is that you are embarrassed to be seen exercising."

If that is the case, then starting your new lifestyle by taking out a membership at the trendy new health club that everyone is going to would probably be a mistake. That membership card will get about as much use as a coupon good for five free wrestling lessons.

Instead, acknowledge your fear and create an environment that guarantees privacy—maybe a stationary bike in your bedroom or an early-morning walk.

The same thing goes for food. If you know in your heart of hearts that you will never give up apple pie, then don't say you will and set yourself up for failure. Create a new recipe that makes apple pie less fattening.

Get support. "If you look at the factors that predict successful, permanent weight loss, social support ranks near the top of the list," says John Foreyt, Ph.D., director of the Nutrition Research Clinic at Baylor College of Medicine in Houston and co-author of *Living without Dieting*. "I'd go so far as to say that it is absolutely critical."

When starting your new lifestyle, Dr. Foreyt insists that you make a public commitment, but not for the normal reasons. "It's not that you want to force yourself into a situation you can't back down from because everyone knows about it. What you are actually doing is making an assertive appeal for people's help and understanding."

In his book, Dr. Foreyt outlines four levels of support, each with its own special purpose. "First there's your family. They're going to need to get used to your new lifestyle. It may be that certain foods have to be kept out of the house. Compromises on family time may need to be made when your exercise or other activities conflict with family plans."

The second level is composed of close friends. "Everyone should have someone they can call when temptation rears its ugly head," says Dr. Foreyt. "Even one really good friend can make the difference in a crisis."

The third and fourth levels involve support groups and your doctor. "Support groups are the perfect place to get advice and encouragement from people experiencing the same things you are," notes Dr. Foreyt. "And your doctor gives you information and feedback and helps you monitor your progress."

For some people, maintaining all four levels of support is not necessary.

But Dr. Foreyt still maintains the need for some form of social support, even for loners. And more important, the kind of support you solicit needs to be specific.

"You don't want people giving you negative support," says Dr. Foreyt. "While someone pointing out your mistakes may work in the short run, it isn't motivating over the long haul. So you want to be very direct about asking people to say something positive about your accomplishments."

Find a monitoring system that works. "Your actual weight is the least important thing you can monitor," says Ronette Kolotkin, Ph.D., director of behavioral programs at Duke University's Diet and Fitness Center and co-author of *The Duke University Medical Center Book of Diet and Fitness*. "Instead, I always encourage people to keep a diary not just of food and exercise but also of any important behavioral problems they encounter, such as rapid eating in certain situations or a tendency to binge at particular times."

At the end of each week, Dr. Kolotkin suggests, study your diary as if you were a weight-loss professional studying someone else's case history. What advice would you give the patient? A one-year follow-up study conducted by Dr. Kolotkin found that people who monitored food intake, exercise and motivation were more successful than those who monitored weight only.

Paying daily homage to the bathroom scale is a dicey proposition for two reasons. First, your body weight is in constant flux. Up a pound today, down two tomorrow. A momentary gain in water weight may have you on the floor in despair despite the fact that the overall picture is improving.

Second, because your new lifestyle of healthy food and exercise is constantly trimming the fat while boosting the lean, a scale may show no change in weight even though you are getting slimmer and more toned by the minute. "That's why I always encourage people to wear form-fitting clothing," says Dr. Kolotkin. "As you lose weight or even as your body composition changes, you'll get feedback every time you need to have your clothes taken in a bit. You'll constantly be aware of what your body is doing by the way your clothes fit."

Plan for trouble. "I always tell people that they can expect to slip," says Dr. Kolotkin. "It will happen. And the difference between moving on and just plain giving up has to do with having some strategy to deal with momentary failure."

There are two ways you don't want to react to a temporary backslide. On one hand, you don't want to be cavalier: "Oh well, I ate that box of doughnuts, but I'll worry about it tomorrow." On the other hand, you don't want to overreact: "Oh no, this is the end! How can I go on after eating my weight in doughnuts? I'm no good."

"You have to be rational," says Dr. Kolotkin. "The first thing to do is acknowledge exactly what happened. 'I was at a party, lost control and ate 5,000 calories.' Don't overemphasize or underemphasize what occurred. Next, put it into perspective. 'Over the past six months, I've made some great changes; I've exercised regularly, eaten right and made serious progress. Compared with what I've achieved, this one incident is hardly a catastrophe. I don't feel great about it, but it isn't the end of the world.'"

Next comes action. A good general doesn't waste time dwelling on defeat. Instead, he immediately plots a course of action that will take him back on the road to victory. "That does not mean you should exercise twice as long tomorrow to make up for today's mistake," says Dr. Kolotkin. "That's a lot like punishing yourself. Instead, you want to take steps to ensure that what happened does not happen again."

If you found yourself bingeing on a bag of chips lying wantonly open in the kitchen, you may want to purge your house of binge foods. If you stopped exercising for a week because of scheduling difficulties, spend some time arranging things so that it doesn't happen again. "Then get right back into your program," says Dr. Kolotkin. "Set two alarm clocks so that you can't avoid waking up and exercising. Meet a friend for lunch who will make sure you eat the right foods. Write out a meal plan."

In other words, make your lifestyle changes foolproof and inescapable for the next few days just to get yourself back on track. Dr. Kolotkin finds that it takes most people only three days to turn around a negative incident.

Learn from past mistakes. What went wrong the last time you tried to lose weight? "When I ask people that, I'll normally get an unproductive answer like they started eating again," says Dr. Kolotkin. "But you need to look at the underlying reasons. Was the diet you placed yourself on too restrictive? Did you find that your meal plans were falling apart because you were often pressed for time and had to eat whatever was available?" Take some time to dig deep and honestly analyze what went wrong.

Create an environment that makes change easy. Weight loss and lifestyle change are so often looked at as matters of sheer willpower. But why make things tough when you can make them easy? "I call it environmental engineering," says Dr. Hanson, "and it's really where you make changes in your environment that make it easier to succeed."

Environmental engineering is a powerful yet simple concept. If you find yourself getting hungry at 3:00 each afternoon and the only thing available is a candy machine down the hall from your office, don't put yourself in the position of having to fight the urge to merge with a chocolate bar. Instead, reach into your desk and pull out the apple that you brought along for just such a moment.

That idea can be applied to all areas of your life. And once you've determined why you've failed in the past, you can set up your new environment to help avoid past mistakes. "When I encounter people who have a problem with after-dinner eating, I often suggest that they get a small refrigerator for beverages and keep it in the den," says Dr. Kolotkin. "That way, even if they are thirsty, they don't need to enter the kitchen and be tempted by an open refrigerator."

As for exercise, did your last walking program peter out after a week because you never seemed to have clean socks, batteries for your personal stereo or rain gear? Get equipped. Keep everything where you can get at it immediately. Keep an extra pair of walking shoes in your car for impromptu opportunities. Make it so easy on yourself that you can't possibly fail.

Take Action

You're ready to get started. But at what pace? Do you purge all the fat from your diet, change your eating habits and throw yourself into a daily exercise program in one fell swoop? Or should you ease into a lifestyle change like you ease into a hot tub—making a few food substitutions, exercising a couple days a week, getting comfortable?

When making your decision, don't think about how fast you want to lose weight. The real question is which technique makes it easier to assimilate changes that you can keep for life.

"If you're looking to make permanent lifestyle changes, my feeling is that incorporating them slowly makes them easier to get used to," says Dr. Kolotkin. "It's less overwhelming. The goals seem more attainable if you go step-by-step rather than full force."

Dr. Kolotkin experienced the power of small changes firsthand in working with a woman who, at age 45, had never exercised and was so out of shape that a flight of stairs would leave her winded and grasping the banister for support. When she started her program, five minutes on a stationary bike was all she could do. "But rather than dwell on the thought that five minutes was not a very big or important change, she embraced the notion of small, gradual changes and took pride in the fact that she was actually exercising at all," says Dr. Kolotkin. "And gradually, over the following months, as she got comfortable with one level of exercise, she increased it. She has now been in four walking marathons!"

Of course, Dr. Kolotkin is quick to admit that gradual change means gradual results, sometimes too gradual for some people. "It's not as exciting or motivating to make small changes, so some people resist it, thinking that they'll never get where they want to be. "But then I remind them that they tried cutting calories too quickly in the past and found the diet too restrictive to continue. Although they did lose some fast weight, in the end, they went back to their old habits and gained it back."

On the other hand, if you like big, exciting changes, you have an ally in Dr. Ornish. According to him, comprehensive changes can make people feel so much better so quickly that, rather than being overwhelmed by the changes, they are instead strongly motivated to continue.

So which is right for you? Part of the answer lies with your doctor and your current situation. Big dietary changes may be within your capability, but if you haven't been exercising regularly, too much activity too fast could be dangerous.

The second part of the answer has to do with your own mental makeup. Do big challenges bring out the best in you or do you find them intimidating? What has worked for you in other situations? Remember, the only right answer here is the one that's right for you.

chapter 2

Best Bets for Health Watchers

EATING LIGHT IN THE REAL WORLD

You're cruising down the interstate when breakfast beckons. It's fast food or nothing, but can you refuel on such fare without taking a detour around your healthy diet?

You're cooling your heels at the airport between flights. Hunger strikes as you catch a whiff of just-baked cookies. A transgression can send you into a tailspin, but can you resist?

Situations like these can be challenging for health-conscious people. But no matter how difficult a situation, choices are usually available—some better than others.

The key in these circumstances is to make choices actively, not passively, says Sachiko St. Jeor, Ph.D., professor of nutrition at the University of Nevada School of Medicine in Reno. "You don't have to be a victim of your environment," Dr. St. Jeor says. "You can take control."

With those words of inspiration in mind, we decided to explore some real diet danger zones to find the best choices. Here are some ideas that may help you make informed food choices in any situation.

Fast-Food Breakfast

GOOD: Pancakes

A decent choice in any fast-food restaurant, assuming you hold the butter or margarine and go easy on the syrup. At Hardee's, which offers the most diet-friendly pancakes by fast-food standards, three pancakes contain 280 calories and just 2 grams of fat (6 percent of calories). McDonald's pancakes aren't bad either, with 245 calories and 4 grams fat (15 percent of calories) in three.

BETTER: McDonald's fat-free apple bran muffin

Only 180 calories, no fat. Add a glass of orange juice (about 60 calories and no fat in 6 ounces) and 8 ounces of 1 percent milk (about 110 calories and 2 grams fat) and you have a pretty nutritious, low-fat breakfast for 350 calories, says Dr. St. Jeor.

BEST: A bowl of nonsugary cereal

McDonald's serves up Cheerios (¾ cup for 80 calories and 1 gram fat) and Wheaties (¾ cup for 90 calories and 1 gram fat)—either of which provides about 15 to 30 percent of the daily quota for iron and vitamins A and C. Pour on the 1 percent milk and the total calorie count is still under 200—plus you meet about a third of your daily calcium requirement.

Fast-Food Chicken Sandwiches

GOOD: Arby's Lite Roast Chicken Deluxe or Wendy's Grilled Chicken Sandwich

Here are two sandwiches worth clucking about. Arby's has 276 calories and 7 grams fat (23 percent of calories). Wendy's chicken sandwich is close, with 290 calories and 7 grams fat (22 percent of calories).

BETTER: Chick-Fil-A Chargrilled Chicken Sandwich

This East Coast chain offers one lean chicken, with just 17 percent of calories from fat (258 calories, 4.8 grams fat). If you have high blood pressure, however, take note: This sandwich may be low in fat, but it's high in sodium, with 1,121 milligrams.

BEWARE: All others

A chicken sandwich by any other name could be a fat trap. Burger King's Chicken Sandwich, for example, will set you back 700 calories, with 54 percent of those calories from fat. McDonald's McChicken (470 calories and 25 grams fat), Wendy's Breaded Chicken (450 calories, 20 grams fat) and Arby's Grilled Chicken Deluxe (430 calories, 19.9 grams fat) aren't much better, with about 40 to 48 percent of calories from fat.

Cinema Fare

OKAY: Red licorice

Red Vines, for example, by American Licorice Company, has only 140 calories and no fat in seven licorice sticks. Trouble is, we're talking empty calories here; red licorice has virtually no nutrient value.

BETTER: Nonbuttered popcorn

Only 55 calories, about 100 milligrams sodium and about 3.1 grams fat per cup for oil-popped corn. The problem is, who can stop at a cup? Most theaters serve up popcorn by the gallon, which makes fat, calorie and sodium totals soar.

BEST: Eat before the film

"Remind yourself that movies last just two hours, and you can go that long without food," says Dr. St. Jeor. "Get into watching the movie as a pure experience, without shoveling down food you can't see or really enjoy."

Midafternoon Snacks

GOOD: Low-fat, low-sugar dried cereal

Cheerios or mini shredded wheat will do. These cereals are not just low in fat but also nutrient-fortified.

ALSO GOOD: Prunes

Seven prunes contain about 140 calories, no fat and 4 grams of dietary fiber.

BEST: Instant bean soup

Packaged in individual serving cups—and available in a wide variety of flavors—instant bean soups are easy to take to the office. Just add boiling water or add cold water and heat in the microwave. Two good choices are a black bean soup made by Fantastic Foods and a couscous tomato minestrone made by Nile Spice. Both are rich and tasty—and can really satisfy an appetite for about 200 calories and 1 gram or less of fat. Nutritionist Evelyn Tribole, R.D., author of *Healthy Homestyle Cooking*, points out that many such soups are high in vitamins (including C and A), minerals like iron, complex carbohydrates and fiber.

Airport Food

GOOD: Sushi

It's becoming as all-American as bagels. In airports, stick with the kind with the cooked fish filling (like those with crabmeat) or vegetable filling to avoid risk of parasites, says Judith S. Stern, Sc.D., professor of nutrition and internal medicine at the University of California, Davis. A full serving of vegetable sushi contains about 365 calories and just 1 gram of fat.

BETTER: Nonfat frozen yogurt

Four ounces of Honey Hill Farms Ghirardelli Chocolate flavor, for example, contains 115 calories, no fat and, as a bonus, 110 milligrams of calcium—a boon for the bones. (Skip the "mix-ins" like chopped candy and nuts.)

EVEN BETTER: A steaming cup of decaf café latte (made with skim milk)

A café latte is mostly hot milk, with a little espresso floated on top. You sate your appetite and do your bones a calcium favor (264 milligrams in 7 ounces for less than 80 calories and less than half a gram of fat).

BEST: Take a fitness walk through the terminal

You can chart your course and ensure that you don't get lost by picking up a map of the terminal at the information desk. Tip: Wear a fanny pack or backpack so you can stride more freely in your travels.

Airplane Meals and Snacks

GOOD: Pasta entrées

Meat entrées are usually greasy, notes Dr. Stern, while pasta entrées are generally lower in fat.

BETTER: Fly American Airlines

They're starting to routinely offer Weight Watchers frozen meals—the same kind you get in the supermarket—on many flights, without advance reservations.

BEST: Plan ahead

Don't leave your in-flight food up to chance. Pack snack food—like fruit, a bagel or serving-size cereal—in your carry-on bag so you won't be tempted by the salted peanuts or smoked almonds, suggests John Foreyt, Ph.D., director of the Nutrition Research Clinic at Baylor College of Medicine in Houston and co-author of *Living without Dieting*. And don't forget to order a special low-fat meal in advance. A low-fat, low-cholesterol breakfast on United Airlines, for example, might include fresh fruit, an asparagus and egg-substitute frittata, mushroom ragout and a roasted tomato half. Talk about friendly skies!

Finally, drink lots of bottled water. It keeps you hydrated and reduces your appetite.

Mixed Drinks

GOOD: Virgin (nonalcoholic) fresh-fruit daiquiris

A daiquiri has about 80 to 100 calories, with little or no fat. The standard recipe calls for about half a cup of fresh fruit (like strawberries, which contain roughly 30 calories), 2 ounces of a mixer called sweet-and-sour (a nonfat lemon-and-sugar drink, with about 50 calories) and a big scoop of ice.

BEST: Virgin Mary

This spicy tomato-juice concoction is a boon in so many ways. It fills you with liquid; it's low-cal—about 32 calories for a 6-ounce glass; it's nonfat; it's spicy, which satisfies tastebuds; it provides some nutrition in the form of vitamin C; and finally, there's a great big celery stick to provide crunch appeal.

Burgers in Disneyland

GOOD: Turkey burger

Served with lettuce, tomato and fat-free Thousand Island dressing on a honey wheat bun, it contains only 367 calories and 9.5 grams fat (23 percent of calories).

BEST: Veggie burger

This burger has the same fat-free dressing and bun as the turkey burger, with only 365 calories and 8 grams fat (19 percent of calories).

Ballpark Fare

GOOD: Check out the latest offerings

It's a whole new ball game out there. Stadium concessionaires are innovating to appeal to the increasing numbers of female sports fans, says Matthew Bauer, media manager for Sportservice Corporation in Buffalo, the leading food supplier to ballparks across the country. Among the new offerings:

- Rotisserie chicken, as an alternative to fried chicken, available at the Texas Rangers Stadium in Arlington. (A great choice, as long as you remove the skin.) Also in several parks: grilled chicken served on a bed of greens.

- The vegetarian burrito at Tiger Stadium in Detroit—loaded with julienned strips of zucchini, peppers and onions in a soft flour tortilla.

- Fresh sliced-turkey sandwiches at Dodger Stadium in Los Angeles and other locales.

- Frozen-fruit pops and low-fat frozen yogurt, available at Sportservice client stadiums, including Milwaukee County Stadium, Riverfront Stadium in Cincinnati, Comiskey Park in Chicago, Busch Stadium in St. Louis and Gateway Stadium in Cleveland.

BEST: Crudités

At Dodger Stadium, they give it a more manly name (relish tray), but that's what it is—a plate loaded with fresh cucumbers, celery, carrots and radishes.

BEWARE: Ordering from your seat

A less-fortunate new trend in stadium cuisine is the legion of waiters sent out with handheld computers who take your order at your seat and then deliver the food to you. Just say no! Stand up and go get it yourself. Walking burns calories.

Chinese Meals

GOOD: A shared entrée of stir-fried vegetables and lots of steamed rice

Chinese-food lovers reeled in shock when news stories revealed that many of their favorite dishes are loaded with fatty oils. And it's true: A typical serving of stir-fried veggies can contain 400 calories and anywhere from 6 to 18 grams of fat. But you can avoid some of the fat and still enjoy this flavorful cuisine by sharing an entrée. To appease your appetite, pile on the steamed rice.

BEST: Steamed veggies with chicken or shrimp

Even if it's not on the menu, most cooks in Chinese restaurants can create a delectable steamed meal. Often, they serve it in a beautiful bamboo steamer. For flavor, sprinkle the food with soy sauce or ask for a brown sauce with scallions on the side to drizzle on top. In these entrées, light-meat chicken contains only about 175 calories and 5 grams fat, while shrimp is even leaner, with only about 85 calories and less than 1 gram of fat.

Restaurant Desserts

GOOD: Two forks

Share whatever dessert you order with a friend. "If you're used to eating dessert and you let yourself have just a bite or two, you'll be less likely to feel deprived and binge later," says Dr. Foreyt.

BETTER: Decaf cappuccino (espresso with frothed skim milk)

Tribole suggests having it with a biscotti or two on the side. Many different companies manufacture biscotti—almond cookies designed for dipping. They're generally low in fat and calories. Some biscotti have only 30 calories and less than 1 gram of fat per cookie.

BEST: Sorbet

This tangy juice-based dessert is mostly water. A half-cup of fruit sorbet, such as pineapple or peach, might provide about 120 calories and no fat.

Chocolate Lovers'
Supermarket Snacks

GOOD: Snackwell's Devil's Food Cookie Cakes

Deep, chocolate, cakey interior surrounded by a thin layer of marshmallow, then a dark chocolate coating—so sweet and rich, it's hard to believe they're fat-free. Drawbacks: Each hefty cookie contains about 50 calories, so you can't eat infinite amounts. They don't really offer vitamins or minerals either. And the leading ingredient is sugar.

ALSO GOOD: Chocolate pudding pops

One pop (made by Jell-O) is only 79 calories, with 2 grams fat.

SPECIAL MENTION: Chocolate-flavored low-fat yogurt

Would you believe chocolate-raspberry yogurt? Chocolate-cherry? Chocolate-cappuccino? They're really, really chocolatey and contain only 200 calories for ¾ cup, with just 2 grams fat. They're put out by Whitney's of New York and are available in some parts of the country.

Seafood Entrées

GOOD: Haddock

Just 112 calories and 1 gram of fat for every 3½ ounces (8 percent of calories from fat).

BEST: Lobster

The winner and still champion. Steamed or boiled, it gets just 5 percent of calories from fat. You get 98 calories and less than a gram of fat in 3½ ounces. You'll need to skip the melted butter, however—try cocktail sauce instead.

BEWARE: Tuna salad

Sorry, Charlie. A cup of tuna salad, with regular mayo, provides 380 calories and 19 grams fat (45 percent of calories).

Munchies

GOOD: Baked Bugles

Unlike the regular Bugles product (with 150 calories and 8 grams of fat per serving), the kind marked "Oven Baked" are relatively low calorie (90 calories for 42 Bugles) and low-fat (2 grams fat). But like the regular product, they taste oily and crunchy. (The sodium is pretty high, though, at 300 milligrams per serving, and they don't offer many nutrients.)

BETTER: Air-popped popcorn

Three cups contain only 93 calories and a gram of fat, plus about 3 grams of dietary fiber.

BETTER YET: Fat-free baked potato chips or tortilla chips

Guiltless Gourmet No-Oil Tortilla Chips contain 110 calories for 22 chips, a respectable 4 grams fiber and zero fat. Similarly, Louise's Fat-Free Potato Chips contain about 100 calories per ounce and no fat.

Beef

GOOD: Healthy Choice Extra-Lean Low-Fat Ground Beef

Four ounces (uncooked) has 4 grams of fat—that's about 28 percent of its calories. By comparison, four ounces of regular ground beef contains 30 grams fat (77 percent of calories).

BETTER: Select-grade top and eye round

With about 20 to 25 percent of calories from fat, they're a cut above all other supermarket-grade cuts.

BEST: New brands of beef that are raised to be low in fat through diet

There are several, including Dakota Lean Meats. Most of the Dakota cuts—ranging from top sirloin to tenderloin to sirloin tips—average about 2.7 grams of fat and 130 calories for every four-ounce serving. That's a respectable 18 percent of calories from fat.

Fun Snacks and Nibbles

SMART CHOICES FOR PARTIES AND BETWEEN MEALS

Americans love to snack, whether it's at a coffee break, after school, at parties or before bedtime. In the 1980s, many of us replaced breakfast, lunch and dinner with more relaxed all-day light eating or snacking and coined a new name for it: "grazing." But traditional party and snack foods are also traditionally high in fat, calories and sodium. Today's grazing requires a healthful, well-balanced "pasture" to browse through. In this chapter, you'll find creative, low-fat appetizers and finger foods to build an elegant party menu, as well as snacks for lunches, outings and casual get-togethers. And all of them will fit into your healthy eating—and easy living—plans.

PREPARATION TIME
10 minutes
plus 10 minutes
marinating time

Vegetarian Spring Rolls

serves 4

Spring rolls are lighter, more delicate uncooked versions of Chinese egg rolls—and the lack of cooking time makes them quicker to prepare.

2	large carrots, julienned
2	tablespoons slivered scallions
$^1/_3$	cup thinly sliced napa cabbage
1	tablespoon olive oil
1	tablespoon minced fresh cilantro
$^1/_4$	teaspoon ground black pepper
1	package (3 ounces) dried bean thread noodles
16	rice-paper rounds (8" size), softened (see note)
2	teaspoons slivered fresh basil or mint
1	tablespoon reduced-sodium soy sauce
1	teaspoon sesame oil

In a large bowl, combine the carrots, scallions, cabbage, olive oil, cilantro and pepper; toss well. Let marinate at room temperature for 10 minutes, stirring frequently.

Place the noodles in a medium bowl. Cover with boiling water and soak for 10 minutes, or until softened. Drain well and snip into 2" pieces.

Place about 2 tablespoons of the noodles and 2 tablespoons of the vegetable mixture on each rice-paper round, about 1" from the lower edge. Sprinkle with the basil or mint. Fold the bottom edge over the filling, fold in both sides and roll up tightly. Press to seal.

In a cup, mix the soy sauce and sesame oil. Serve as a dipping sauce with the spring rolls.

Chef's Note

To soften the rice-paper rounds before rolling them, fill a large bowl with warm water. Dip each round into the water for 10 seconds, or until translucent. Let drain on a clean dish towel. (Do not stack the rice papers or they will stick together.)

Fun Snacks and Nibbles

Artichoke and Leek Pizzas

makes 4

PER PIZZA

354 calories

5.6 g. fat
(14% of calories)

3.4 g. dietary fiber

8 mg. cholesterol

486 mg. sodium

Native to the Mediterranean countries, the leek has been prized by cooks for centuries. This recipe blends the leek's mellow flavor with another Mediterranean favorite, artichoke hearts.

1	turkey bacon strip, chopped
1/2	onion, finely chopped
1	can (14 ounces) artichoke hearts, drained and coarsely chopped
1	large leek, thinly sliced
	Salt and ground black pepper
	Pizza dough (see note)
1/4	cup shredded part-skim mozzarella cheese
2	tablespoons grated Parmesan cheese

PREPARATION TIME
20 minutes

BAKING TIME
10 minutes

In a large no-stick frying pan, cook the bacon for 3 minutes, or until golden; drain on paper towels. Wipe the pan with a paper towel. Add the onions and cook for 3 minutes, or until soft but not brown. Stir in the artichokes, leeks and bacon. Season with the salt and pepper.

Coat a large baking sheet with no-stick spray. Divide the dough into 4 pieces; form into 6" rounds and place on the sheet.

Top with the artichoke mixture and sprinkle with the mozzarella and Parmesan.

Bake at 500° for 10 minutes, or until the bottoms are crisp and brown.

Chef's Note

To make pizza dough: In a food processor, combine 1 3/4 cups all-purpose flour, 1 tablespoon rye flour, 1 tablespoon cornmeal, 1 package quick-rise yeast, 1/2 teaspoon salt and 1/2 teaspoon sugar. With the motor running, add 3/4 cup warm water (about 125°) and 1 1/2 teaspoons olive oil. Process until a ball forms, then process for 1 minute to knead. Let rest for 10 minutes.

PREPARATION TIME
15 minutes

COOKING TIME
12 minutes

Caponata

serves 4

Serve this eggplant mixture on bruschetta or lettuce leaves. You can easily make this ahead—and, in fact, the flavor actually improves if you let it stand at least 2 hours.

1	teaspoon olive oil
1	eggplant, peeled and cut into 1" cubes
1	cup chopped tomatoes
1	sweet red pepper, coarsely chopped
1	green pepper, coarsely chopped
1	onion, coarsely chopped
3	cloves garlic, minced
15	black olives, pitted and chopped
¼	cup drained capers
¼	cup chopped fresh parsley
2	tablespoons chopped fresh marjoram
1	tablespoon red wine vinegar

Warm the oil in a large no-stick frying pan over medium-high heat. Add the eggplant and sauté for 2 minutes. Add the tomatoes, red peppers, green peppers, onions and garlic. Reduce the heat and simmer for 10 minutes, stirring occasionally. Stir in the olives, capers, parsley, marjoram and vinegar.

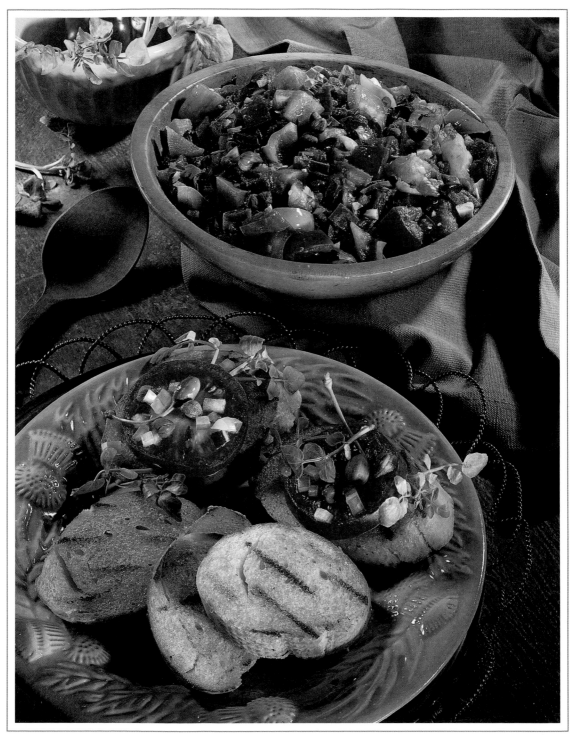

Bruschetta recipe on page 38

PREPARATION TIME
5 minutes

BAKING TIME
5 minutes

Photo on page 37

Bruschetta

makes 4

Bruschetta are simple garlic toasts that can be served unadorned or with fresh toppings.

> 4   slices Italian or sourdough bread
>
> 2   cloves garlic, halved lengthwise
>
> 1   tablespoon olive oil

Place the bread on a baking sheet and broil about 5" from the heat until lightly toasted on both sides. While still hot, rub one side of each slice with the garlic, pressing the juice into the toast. Using a brush, spread the oil over the garlic side of the toast.

VARIATIONS

Tomato and Watercress Bruschetta

Layer 4 bruschetta with 1 cup watercress leaves and tomato slices. Sprinkle with ¼ cup chopped red onions, 1 tablespoon drained capers and 1 teaspoon olive oil.

PER SERVING: 143 calories, 4.6 g. fat (30% of calories), 1.6 g. dietary fiber, 0 mg. fiber, 190 mg. sodium

Cucumber, Sun-Dried Tomato and Olive Bruschetta

Layer 4 bruschetta with 1 small cucumber (peeled, seeded and thinly sliced). Top with sun-dried tomato halves (soaked in hot water, drained and chopped). Sprinkle with 2 tablespoons chopped black olives and 2 tablespoons chopped fresh basil.

PER SERVING: 142 calories, 4.2 g. fat (26% of calories), 1.9 g. dietary fiber, 0 mg. fiber, 177 mg. sodium

White Bean
and Roasted Garlic Spread

makes 3 cups

Serve this flavorful mixture as a spread on toast triangles or crackers. Or use it as a stuffing for celery pieces, hollowed-out cherry tomatoes or Belgian endive leaves.

PER 2 TABLESPOONS

40 calories

0.7 g. fat
(16% of calories)

1 g. dietary fiber

0 mg. fiber

1 mg. sodium

1	garlic bulb
2	cans (19 ounces each) white beans, rinsed and drained
1/4	cup lemon juice
1	tablespoon olive oil
2	tablespoons minced fresh parsley
1/4	teaspoon ground black pepper
1/4	cup minced red onions
1/4	cup minced green peppers

PREPARATION TIME
10 minutes

BAKING TIME
15 minutes

Break the garlic bulb into cloves. Place the unpeeled cloves in a custard cup and cover with aluminum foil. Bake at 400° for 15 minutes, or until soft when tested with the tip of a knife. Do not allow the garlic to brown. Let cool slightly, then slip off the skins and trim off the hard stem ends.

Place half of the beans in a food processor. Add the lemon juice, oil and garlic. Process until smooth. Transfer to a medium bowl. Stir in the parsley, black pepper, half of the onions, half of the green peppers and the remaining beans. Roughly mash the whole beans with a fork.

Sprinkle with the remaining onions and green peppers.

PREPARATION TIME
20 minutes

BAKING TIME
5 minutes

Twice-Baked New Potatoes

serves 8

Low-fat dairy products are the key to slimming down this party favorite.

4   medium new potatoes

2   tablespoons minced onions

3   tablespoons fat-free sour cream

1   tablespoon finely shredded reduced-fat Cheddar cheese
     Pinch of ground black pepper

$1/4$ teaspoon crushed pink peppercorns

Pierce the potatoes in several places with a fork and microwave on high power for 7 to 10 minutes (turning once), or until the potatoes are tender. Let stand for 5 minutes, or until cool enough to handle.

Coat a small no-stick frying pan with no-stick spray. Place over medium heat until hot. Add the onions and sauté for 3 to 4 minutes, or until lightly browned.

Cut the potatoes lengthwise into quarters and scoop out the centers with a spoon, leaving $1/4$"-thick shells. Place the centers in a medium bowl and mash with a potato masher or fork. Stir in the onions, sour cream, Cheddar and black pepper. Pipe or spoon into the potato shells.

Place the potatoes on a large baking sheet and bake at 475° for 3 to 5 minutes, or until the filling is hot. Top with the peppercorns.

Fun Snacks and Nibbles

Pita Party Pizza

makes 16 slices

Pita rounds make perfect instant pizza crusts. The feta cheese, spinach and olives give this pizza Greek flair.

PER SLICE

32 calories

0.7 g. fat
(19% of calories)

0.8 g. dietary fiber

1 mg. fiber

52 mg. sodium

2	whole-wheat pita breads
1	box (10 ounces) frozen chopped spinach, thawed and squeezed dry
1/2	cup shredded fat-free mozzarella cheese
1/4	cup crumbled feta cheese
1/4	cup sliced black olives
1	tomato, chopped
1/4	cup thinly sliced red onions

PREPARATION TIME
10 minutes

BAKING TIME
10 minutes

Prick the pitas several times with a fork. Spread the spinach over the pitas. Sprinkle with the mozzarella, feta, olives, tomatoes and onions. Place the pitas on a baking sheet and bake at 400° for 10 minutes.

To serve, cut each pizza into 8 slices.

PREPARATION TIME
10 minutes

COOKING TIME
15 minutes

Light 'n' Lean Nachos

serves 8

Nachos are a perennial favorite, but they're generally loaded with fat, sodium and calories. In this healthier version, potatoes replace the traditional deep-fried tortilla chips.

1½	pounds large potatoes, scrubbed and sliced crosswise ⅜" thick
½	cup defatted chicken broth
1⅓	cups salsa
1	cup rinsed and drained canned pinto or white beans
½	teaspoon hot-pepper sauce
⅔	cup shredded reduced-fat Monterey Jack cheese

In a 4-cup glass measuring cup, combine half of the potatoes and ¼ cup of the broth. Cover with vented plastic wrap and microwave on high power for 5 to 7 minutes, or until the potatoes are just tender.

Let stand for 5 minutes, or until cool enough to handle. Drain the potatoes and pat them dry with paper towels. Spread on a large microwave-safe serving plate.

In a small bowl, mix the salsa, beans and hot-pepper sauce. Spoon half of the mixture over the potatoes. Sprinkle with ⅓ cup of the Monterey Jack. Loosely cover with wax paper.

Microwave on medium (50% power) for 2 minutes, or until the cheese has melted. Serve immediately.

Repeat with the remaining potatoes, broth, salsa mixture and Monterey Jack.

Chef's Notes

Microwaving cheese on medium power prevents it from turning rubbery.

If you don't have a microwave, steam the potato slices until tender, about 10 minutes. Then spread them on ovenproof platters and top with the salsa mixture and cheese. Bake at 350° for 15 minutes.

Festive Kabobs

makes 8

Your guests will relish these colorful tortellini skewers.

PER KABOB

117 calories

2.4 g. fat
(18% of calories)

0.8 g. dietary fiber

10 mg. fiber

110 mg. sodium

16	cheese-filled spinach tortellini
8	cheese-filled white tortellini
⅔	cup fat-free Italian dressing
¼	cup water
16	cherry tomatoes
8	small mushrooms
16	pieces (1" × 1") yellow peppers
16	pieces (1" × 1") sweet red peppers
8	pieces (1" × 1") green peppers
¼	teaspoon olive oil

PREPARATION TIME
5 minutes
plus chilling time

COOKING TIME
10 minutes

Cook the tortellini in a large pot of boiling water according to the package directions. Drain and place in a large shallow baking dish.

In a small bowl, whisk together the dressing and water. Pour over the tortellini. Add the tomatoes and mushrooms. Stir to coat.

In a 1-quart microwave-safe casserole, mix the yellow peppers, red peppers, green peppers and oil. Cover with vented plastic wrap and microwave on high power for 2 to 4 minutes, or until the peppers are crisp-tender. Add to the baking dish. Toss gently. Chill.

Evenly divide the ingredients among 8 wooden skewers.

Cocktail Meatballs Florentine

serves 8

Spinach and cheese are what make these versatile and delicious meatballs "florentine." Serve with warmed marinara sauce or salsa for additional flavor.

8	cloves garlic, unpeeled
1	teaspoon olive oil
4	shallots
1	cup fresh spinach leaves
$1/2$	cup fat-free ricotta cheese
1	egg white
2	teaspoons dried oregano
$1/2$	teaspoon ground black pepper
$1/2$	teaspoon dried dill
$1/4$	teaspoon ground nutmeg
12	ounces extra-lean ground beef
$1/3$	cup fresh whole-wheat bread crumbs

Combine the garlic and oil in a custard cup, cover with aluminum foil and bake at 400° for 15 minutes, or until soft when tested with the tip of a knife. Do not allow the garlic to brown. Let cool slightly, then slip off the skins and trim off the hard stem ends.

In a food processor, puree the garlic, shallots, spinach, ricotta and egg white. Add the oregano, pepper, dill and nutmeg.

In a large bowl, combine the beef and bread crumbs. Add the spinach mixture and mix well.

Shape into 32 meatballs. Line a jelly-roll pan with aluminum foil. Place a wire rack on the foil. Coat the rack with no-stick spray. Place the meatballs on the rack and bake at 400° for 20 to 25 minutes, or until brown.

Fun Snacks and Nibbles

Spicy Garlic Bread

makes 16 slices

PER SLICE

106 calories

4.6 g. fat
(39% of calories)

0.8 g. dietary fiber

1 mg. fiber

182 mg. sodium

Ground red pepper adds zip to this flavorful bread. Olive oil trims the saturated fat to zero.

¼	cup olive oil
3	cloves garlic, minced
1	loaf French bread, cut in half lengthwise
¼	cup shredded Parmesan cheese
¼	teaspoon ground red pepper

PREPARATION TIME
5 minutes

BAKING TIME
4 minutes

In a small bowl, mix the oil and garlic. Spread onto the cut sides of the bread. Sprinkle with the Parmesan and pepper.

Place, cut side up, on a baking sheet and broil about 4" from the heat for 3 to 4 minutes, or until lightly browned. Cut into 16 slices.

Herbed Crouton Toasts

makes 8

This simple bread is so delicious you will serve it often. It is particularly good with soups and stews. For variety, use other herbs, like marjoram, basil or oregano.

8   thick slices French or Italian bread

1   tablespoon dried thyme

   Salt and ground black pepper

Arrange the bread on a large baking sheet. Coat each slice with no-stick spray; sprinkle with the thyme, salt and pepper. Bake at 400° for 15 minutes, or until crisp and golden brown.

Photo on page 69

Red Pepper–Ricotta Bruschetta

makes 8

8   thick slices French bread

1/2   cup reduced-fat ricotta cheese

2   tablespoons fat-free mayonnaise

2   tablespoons fat-free plain yogurt

2   tablespoons grated Parmesan cheese

1   jar (3 1/2 ounces) chopped roasted sweet red peppers, drained

Toast the bread.

In a small bowl, mix the ricotta, mayonnaise, yogurt and Parmesan. Spread on the toasted bread. Top with the red peppers.

Pita Chips

serves 8

Perfect for dipping, these zesty chips are a delicious, low-fat substitute for potato and corn chips.

PER SERVING

97 calories

2.1 g. fat
(20% of calories)

0.5 g. dietary fiber

0 mg. fiber

187 mg. sodium

PREPARATION TIME
10 minutes

BAKING TIME
10 minutes

6	pita breads
1	tablespoon olive oil
1	tablespoon butter-flavored sprinkles
1/2	teaspoon dried oregano
1/4	teaspoon ground black pepper
1/4	teaspoon chili powder

Cut each pita in half crosswise. Then carefully separate each half into 2 semicircles by cutting open the closed edge.

In a cup, combine the oil, sprinkles, oregano, pepper and chili powder. Lightly brush the interior side of each pita with the mixture. Cut each piece into 4 wedges.

Arrange the chips in a single layer on large baking sheets. Bake at 375° for 5 to 10 minutes, or until crisped. Serve warm.

Chef's Note

If preparing just a portion of the chips, you may microwave them. Line a large microwave–safe plate with a paper towel. Arrange 16 wedges at a time around the outer edge of the plate with the points facing inward. Microwave on high power for 2 minutes. Rotate the plate a half turn. Microwave for 1 to 2 minutes, or until the wedges begin to curl and brown.

PREPARATION TIME
10 minutes

Seven-Layer Skinny Dip

serves 20

*Seven-layer dip always makes a big hit at parties, and this low-fat version
will be equally popular. Serve it with homemade tortilla chips for "scooping."*

1	can fat-free refried beans
1	cup fat-free sour cream
1/2	cup fat-free mayonnaise
1	teaspoon chili powder
1	teaspoon ground cumin
1	cup shredded fat-free Cheddar cheese
1/2	cup chopped scallions
1/2	cup sliced black olives
1	tomato, chopped
1/2	avocado, chopped

Spread the refried beans over the bottom of a 9" pie plate. In a small bowl,
mix the sour cream, mayonnaise, chili powder and cumin. Spread over the
beans. Sprinkle with the Cheddar, scallions, olives, tomatoes and avocados.

Chef's Note

For easy homemade fat-free refried beans, rinse and drain your favorite
canned beans and mash them with a fork or in a food processor.

Fresh Tomato Salsa with Homemade Tortilla Chips recipe on page 56

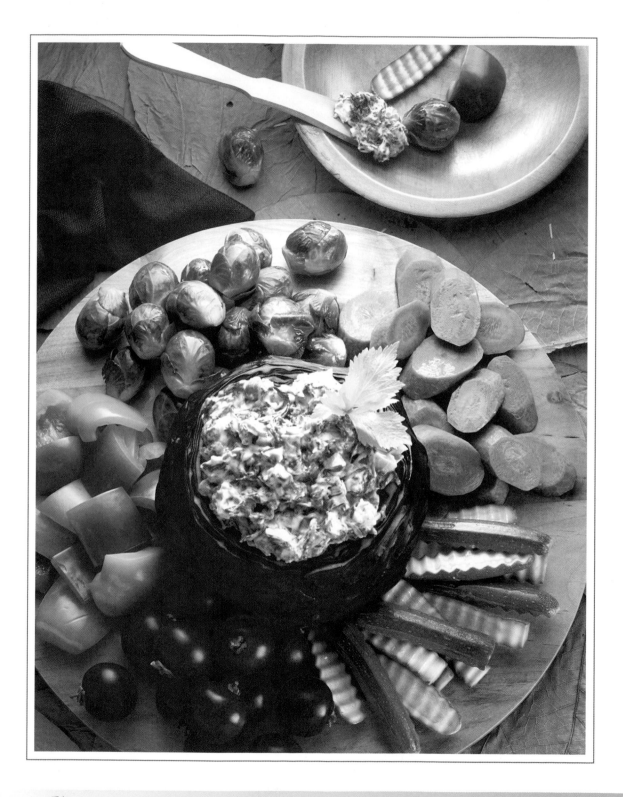

Spinach Dip

serves 8

This dip is particularly easy. But do allow at least 30 minutes for the yogurt to drain so the dip will be nice and thick. If you're not fond of lots of garlic, use only one or two cloves. Serve with crisp fresh vegetables.

PER SERVING

57 calories

1.9 g. fat
(30% of calories)

0.6 g. dietary fiber

0.3 mg. fiber

63 mg. sodium

2	cups fat-free plain yogurt
1	tablespoon olive oil
4	cloves garlic, minced
1	cup packed fresh spinach, finely chopped
1/4	teaspoon lemon juice
1/8	teaspoon ground black pepper

PREPARATION TIME
5 minutes
plus 30 minutes
draining time

COOKING TIME
5 minutes

Spoon the yogurt into a yogurt cheese funnel or a sieve lined with cheesecloth. Place over a bowl and allow to drain for 30 minutes.

Warm the oil in a large no-stick frying pan over medium heat. Add the garlic and cook, stirring constantly, for 1 minute. Add the spinach. Cook, stirring, for 2 minutes, or until wilted. Remove from the heat.

Stir in the yogurt, lemon juice and pepper. Transfer to a shallow serving dish.

PREPARATION TIME
10 minutes

BAKING TIME
10 minutes

Photo on page 53

Fresh Tomato Salsa with Homemade Tortilla Chips

serves 8

Goat cheese gives this traditional salsa an unexpected flavor twist. Enjoy it with these easy-to-make tortilla chips.

1	cup chopped plum tomatoes
1/2	cup chopped scallions
1/2	cup chopped fresh coriander
1	tablespoon grated lime rind
1	tablespoon lime juice
1	teaspoon olive oil
1/2	jalapeño pepper, seeded and minced (wear plastic gloves when handling)
1	tablespoon crumbled goat cheese
4	large flour tortillas

In a medium bowl, mix the tomatoes, scallions, coriander, lime rind, lime juice, oil and peppers. Sprinkle with the goat cheese.

Cut each tortilla into 8 wedges. Coat a large baking sheet with no-stick spray. Place the wedges on the sheet. Bake at 350° for 10 minutes, or until golden and crispy. Serve with the salsa.

Chef's Note

Plum tomatoes are small and meaty with less juice and fewer seeds than regular tomatoes. They're often called Italian tomatoes or Roma tomatoes.

Potato Chips

serves 4

It's easy to make your own healthy chips. For nice thin ones, use a manual slicing machine (inexpensive plastic ones are available at cooking stores). For a gourmet touch, try blue or purple potatoes.

2   Idaho potatoes

2   sweet potatoes

Slice the potatoes as thin as possible (about 20 slices per potato). Place 10 slices at a time on a microwave-safe rack and microwave on high power for 4 minutes, or until golden and crispy.

Watch the first batch carefully; microwaving time depends on the moisture content of the potatoes. If after 4 minutes the potatoes are not crisp, continue microwaving for 30 seconds at a time. Repeat to cook all the slices.

Chef's Note

If you don't have a microwave, place a wire rack on a baking sheet. Arrange the potato slices on the rack. Bake at 450° for 15 to 20 minutes.

PER SERVING

66 calories

0.1 g. fat
(1% of calories)

1.8 g. dietary fiber

0 mg. fiber

5 mg. sodium

PREPARATION TIME
5 minutes

COOKING TIME
40 minutes

Photo on page 58

Potato Chips recipe on page 57; Tangy Eggplant Dip recipe on page 60

Red Pepper Dip

makes 1 cup

Roasted red peppers give this dip an intriguing smoky-sweet flavor. Use fresh vegetables, pita chips or homemade potato chips as dippers.

1	jar (7 ounces) roasted sweet red peppers, drained
½	cup fat-free cream cheese
2	scallions, coarsely chopped
1	clove garlic, coarsely chopped
1	tablespoon lemon juice

Place the peppers, cream cheese, scallions, garlic and lemon juice in a blender or food processor. Process until pureed.

PREPARATION TIME
15 minutes

COOKING TIME
20 minutes

Photo on page 58

Tangy Eggplant Dip

makes 3⅓ cups

Serve on bruschetta or use as a great pasta sauce.

1   eggplant, peeled and finely chopped

1   cup minced onions

1   cup finely chopped celery

1   teaspoon olive oil

1   can (14½ ounces) stewed tomatoes

2   tablespoons red wine vinegar

2   tablespoons currants

1   tablespoon drained capers

In a large no-stick frying pan over medium heat, sauté the eggplant, onions and celery in the oil for 5 minutes, or until soft and lightly browned. Add the tomatoes and break them into small pieces with a spoon. Stir in the vinegar, currants and capers. Reduce the heat to low and cook for 15 minutes.

Middle Eastern Chick-Pea Dip

makes 2 cups

Serve this version of hummus with warm pita wedges that you can use to scoop up the dip.

PREPARATION TIME
10 minutes

1	can (16 ounces) chick-peas, rinsed and drained
½	cup fat-free yogurt
¼	cup minced scallions
¼	cup packed fresh parsley, minced
	Juice of 2 lemons
5	teaspoons tahini
3	cloves garlic, minced
⅛	teaspoon ground black pepper
	Dash of reduced-sodium soy sauce
	Pinch of ground red pepper

In a food processor, process the chick-peas until smooth, stopping to scrape down the sides of the container as necessary.

Add the yogurt, scallions, parsley, lemon juice, tahini, garlic, black pepper, soy sauce and red pepper. Process until smooth and creamy. (If necessary, add a few teaspoons of water to achieve the proper consistency.)

Spread in an even layer on a large shallow platter. If not serving immediately, cover and chill. Serve at room temperature for best flavor.

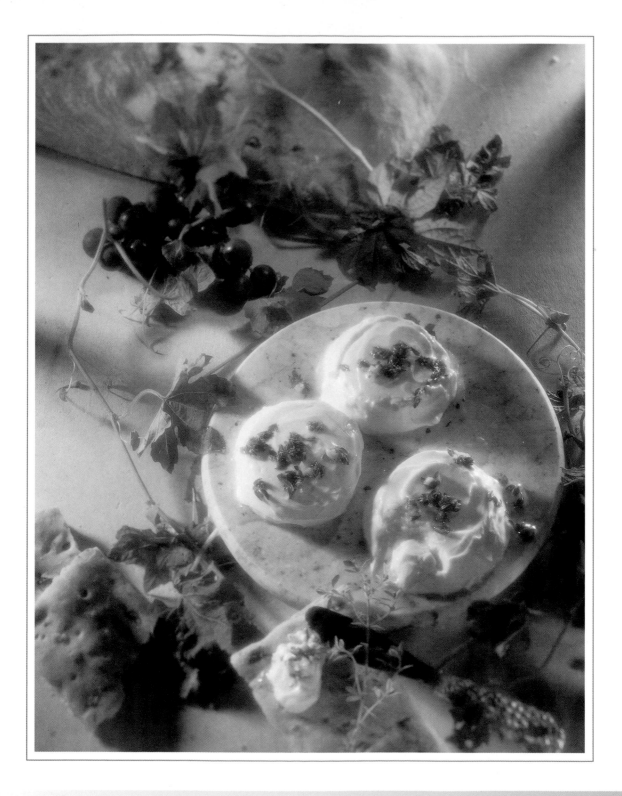

Herb-Garlic Yogurt Cheese

makes 2 cups

Serve this tangy yogurt cheese with crusty bread, crostini or crackers. It's also good on baked potatoes.

1	cup yogurt cheese (see note)
2	teaspoons olive oil
1	teaspoon lemon juice
1	teaspoon chopped fresh thyme
1	teaspoon chopped fresh parsley
1	clove garlic, minced
	Salt and ground black pepper

Divide the yogurt cheese into 4 rounds, flattening them lightly with your palms. Place in a wide, shallow bowl.

In a small bowl, whisk together the oil, lemon juice, thyme, parsley and garlic; add salt and pepper to taste. Pour over the rounds. Let marinate at room temperature for at least 30 minutes before serving.

Chef's Notes

To make the yogurt cheese, spoon 2 cups fat-free plain yogurt into a yogurt cheese funnel or a sieve lined with cheesecloth. Place over a bowl. Cover, refrigerate and allow to drain for 8 hours, or until very thick.

The longer the yogurt cheese marinates, the more flavorful it will be. It will keep, covered, in the refrigerator for 2 days. Allow it to come to room temperature before serving.

PREPARATION TIME
5 minutes
plus 30 minutes
marinating time

PREPARATION TIME
10 minutes

Lime Dip with Fresh Fruit

serves 4

Fresh fruit makes a lovely appetizer. In this recipe, it's served with a creamy sweet-tart dressing that's fat-free. You may substitute other fruit according to what's in season.

¼ cup fat-free mayonnaise

¼ cup fat-free sour cream

Grated rind of 1 lime

3 tablespoons lime juice

2 tablespoons honey

1 bunch red grapes

2 oranges, cut into wedges

In a small bowl, whisk together the mayonnaise, sour cream, lime rind, lime juice and honey. Place in the center of a platter and surround with the grapes and oranges.

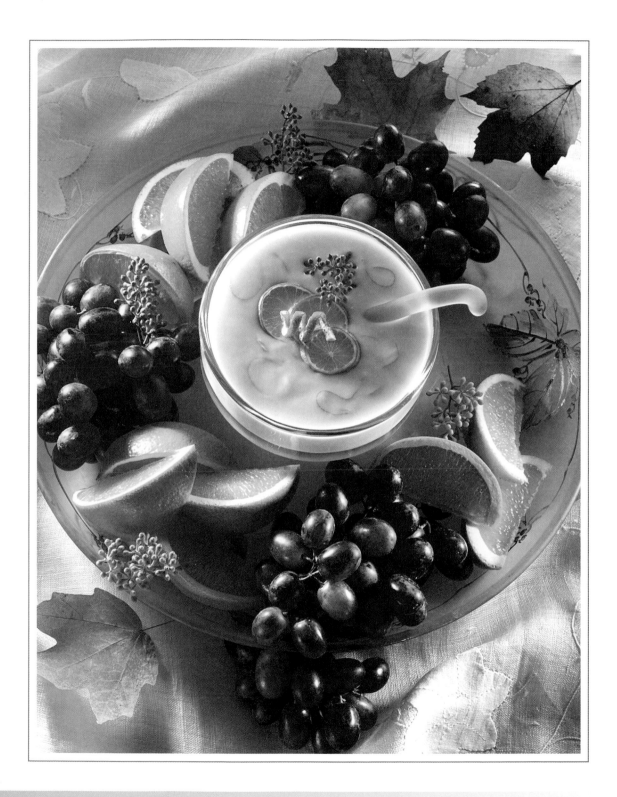

chapter 4

Soups and Salads

OLD FAVORITES . . . AND LOTS MORE

*E*ach region of America boasts an incredible variety of fruits, vegetables, meat, poultry and seafood that have been adopted and adapted by the immigrants who settled this country. In the East, they dreamed up new ways to use clams and oysters; in the North, they turned to the Ojibwa for wild rice. The South melded the sweet and spicy flavors of the Caribbean with European dishes; in the West, they capitalized on a garden of fresh fruits and vegetables. And in the Southwest, they adopted fiery chili peppers to season dishes of all types. The soups and salads in this chapter make the most of regional ingredients and reflect America's ethnic diversity.

Butternut Squash Bisque

serves 4

This simple soup is a fast and delicious way to incorporate high beta-carotene butternut squash into your meals.

1	large butternut squash
1	teaspoon olive oil
2¼	cups defatted chicken broth
2	cups chopped onions
1	cup chopped sweet red peppers
2	teaspoons minced garlic
¼–½	teaspoon ground red pepper
½	teaspoon ground cumin
	Salt and ground black pepper
¼	cup fat-free plain yogurt

Pierce the squash several times with a sharp knife; place it on a paper towel in the microwave. Microwave on high power for 5 minutes. Halve the squash lengthwise and remove and discard the seeds; microwave for 5 minutes.

In a large saucepan over medium-high heat, combine the oil and ¼ cup of the broth; bring to a boil. Add the onions, red peppers and garlic; cook, stirring often, for 5 minutes.

Scoop the squash from its shell and cut into chunks. Add the squash, ground red pepper, cumin and the remaining 2 cups broth to the pan. Cover and bring to a boil. Reduce the heat and simmer for 15 minutes.

Working in batches, transfer the soup to a blender or food processor; process until smooth. Return the soup to the pan; heat through. Add salt and black pepper to taste. Serve garnished with the yogurt.

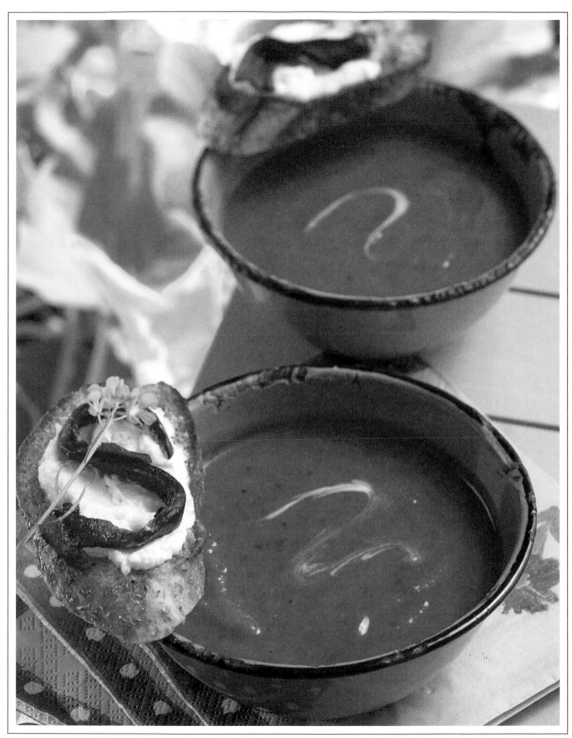

Red Pepper–Ricotta Bruschetta recipe on page 50

PREPARATION TIME
5 minutes

COOKING TIME
20 minutes

White Bean Soup with Basil and Tomatoes

serves 4

A surprisingly light yet satisfying soup, this is best in the summer when fresh basil and tomatoes are at their peak.

1/4	cup chopped onions
1	clove garlic, minced
1/2	teaspoon olive oil
2	cups defatted chicken broth
2	cups water
1	can (15 ounces) navy or cannellini beans, rinsed and drained
1	large potato, peeled and diced
1	teaspoon chopped fresh oregano
	Salt and ground black pepper
1/4	cup finely chopped tomatoes
2	tablespoons chopped fresh basil

In a large saucepan over medium heat, sauté the onions and garlic in the oil for 1 minute. Add the broth, water, beans, potatoes and oregano. Cover and bring to a boil. Reduce the heat and simmer for 15 minutes, or until the potatoes are tender.

Puree about three-fourths of the soup in a blender or food processor. Pour the puree back into the pot and heat through. Add salt and pepper to taste. Stir in the tomatoes and basil.

Chef's Note

In the winter, substitute chopped reconstituted sun-dried tomatoes for the fresh tomatoes and fresh parsley for the basil.

Panzanella recipe on page 96

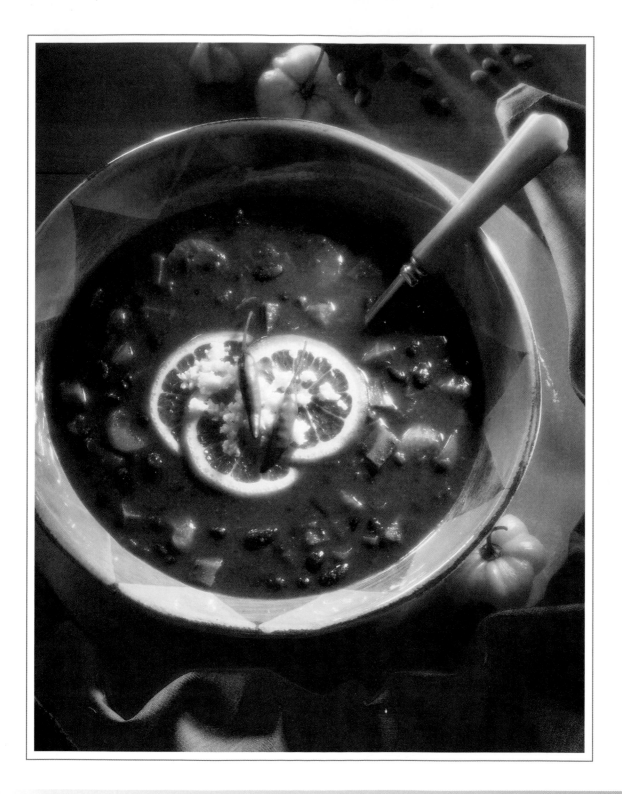

Miami Black Bean Soup

serves 4

This thick, spicy soup reflects its Caribbean heritage with cumin, red-pepper flakes and jalapeño peppers.

PER SERVING

244 calories

3.6 g. fat
(11% of calories)

14.6 g. dietary fiber

0 mg. cholesterol

960 mg. sodium

1½	cups diced onions
2	stalks celery, diced
2	carrots, diced
4	cloves garlic, minced
1	teaspoon olive oil
3	cans (15 ounces each) black beans, rinsed and drained
2½	cups defatted chicken broth
2	cups canned crushed tomatoes
1½	tablespoons lime juice
1½	teaspoons ground cumin
½	teaspoon red-pepper flakes
⅓	cup fat-free sour cream
⅓	cup diced sweet red, yellow or green peppers
2	tablespoons sliced jalapeño peppers (wear plastic gloves when handling)

PREPARATION TIME
10 minutes

COOKING TIME
25 minutes

In a large saucepan over medium heat, sauté the onions, celery, carrots and garlic in the oil for 3 to 4 minutes, or until the vegetables begin to soften. Add the beans, broth, tomatoes, lime juice, cumin and red-pepper flakes. Cover and bring to a boil. Reduce the heat and simmer for 15 to 20 minutes, or until the vegetables are tender.

Serve garnished with the sour cream, sweet peppers and jalapeño peppers.

Minestrone

serves 4

<table>
<tr><td>PER SERVING</td></tr>
<tr><td>240 calories</td></tr>
<tr><td>3.4 g. fat
(12% of calories)</td></tr>
<tr><td>9.4 g. dietary fiber</td></tr>
<tr><td>0 mg. cholesterol</td></tr>
<tr><td>609 mg. sodium</td></tr>
</table>

PREPARATION TIME
15 minutes

COOKING TIME
35 minutes

In Italy, minestrone ("big soup") means just about any kind of soup made with pasta, beans and whatever vegetables are growing in the garden. In winter, it's made with canned tomatoes and root vegetables. As with most soups, reheating heightens the flavors. This recipe is easily doubled so you can have extra to freeze.

1	cup chopped onions
1	clove garlic, minced
½	teaspoon olive oil
2	cups shredded cabbage
1	cup sliced carrots
1	cup chopped spinach
½	cup sliced celery
½	cup chopped fresh parsley
2	bay leaves
2	teaspoons chopped fresh rosemary
1	teaspoon chopped fresh sage
2	cups defatted chicken broth
2	cups water
1	can (15 ounces) no-salt-added stewed tomatoes, chopped (with juice)
1	can (16 ounces) chick-peas, rinsed and drained
4	ounces spaghetti, broken in half
	Salt and ground black pepper

In a large soup pot over medium-high heat, sauté the onions and garlic in the oil for 1 minute. Add the cabbage, carrots, spinach, celery, parsley, bay leaves, rosemary and sage; sauté for 3 minutes, or until the vegetables begin to wilt. Add the broth, water, tomatoes (with juice), chick-peas and spaghetti. Cover and bring to a boil. Reduce the heat and simmer for 20 minutes. Uncover and cook for 10 minutes. Remove and discard the bay leaves. Add salt and pepper to taste.

Chef's Note
For a thinner soup, add up to 4 cups broth.

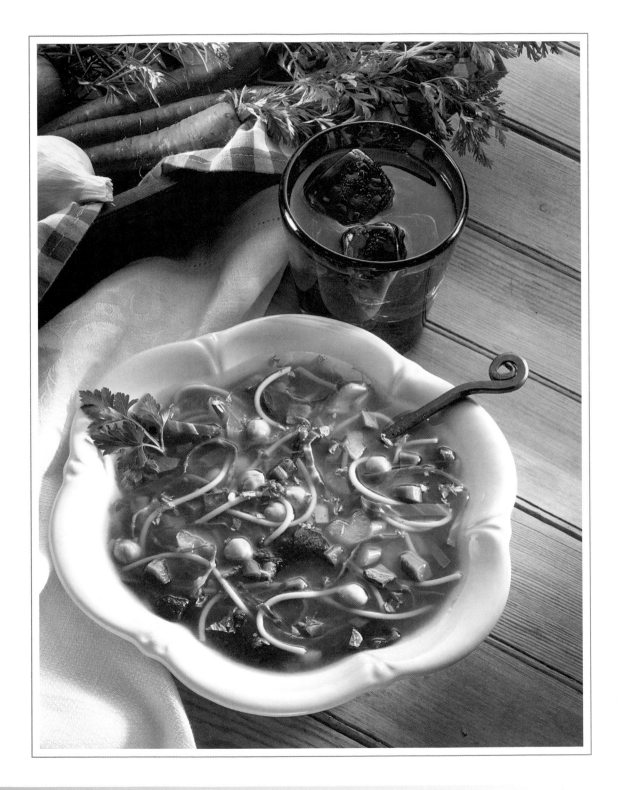

PER SERVING

273 calories

7.4 g. fat
(24% of calories)

2.4 g. dietary fiber

43 mg. cholesterol

104 mg. sodium

PREPARATION TIME
10 minutes

COOKING TIME
25 minutes

Vibrant Chicken and Rice Soup

serves 6

Who doesn't love chicken and rice soup? This variation has a California flavor, featuring avocado, coriander and lime juice as accents.

4	cups water
2	cups defatted chicken broth
1	onion, diced
3	carrots, thinly sliced
3	boneless, skinless chicken breast halves, cubed
2½	cups cooked rice
1	small avocado, cubed
2	tomatoes, cubed
3	tablespoons minced fresh coriander
3	tablespoons lime juice
⅛	teaspoon ground red pepper
4	ounces farmer's cheese, crumbled

In a large soup pot over medium heat, bring the water, broth, onions and carrots to a boil. Reduce the heat and simmer for 10 minutes. Add the chicken and simmer for 10 minutes, or until the chicken is cooked through and the carrots are tender.

Stir in the rice, avocados, tomatoes, coriander, lime juice and pepper. Heat through but don't boil. Serve sprinkled with the farmer's cheese.

Quick Oyster Stew

serves 4

Oysters are good sources of important minerals, including iron and zinc. They even contain a fair share of copper, which helps regulate cholesterol metabolism. For those reasons alone, they would rate a place in your diet. But they're also delicious and make a wonderful chowder.

1	onion, minced
1	stalk celery, minced
1	tablespoon olive oil
1	clove garlic, minced
$1/2$	teaspoon dried savory
1	baking potato, diced
$1^1/2$	cups defatted chicken broth
$1/2$	cup bottled clam juice
$1/2$	cup corn
$1^1/2$	cups small oysters, drained
$1^1/2$	cups 1% low-fat milk
$1/4$	cup minced fresh parsley

In a large saucepan over medium heat, sauté the onions and celery in the oil for 5 minutes, or until tender. Add the garlic and savory; stir for 30 seconds.

Add the potatoes, broth and clam juice. Cover and bring to a boil. Reduce the heat and simmer for 15 minutes, or until the potatoes are tender.

Stir in the corn and oysters. Simmer over low heat for 5 minutes, or until the oysters are just cooked through and their edges have begun to curl. Add the milk and parsley; heat briefly.

PER SERVING

266 calories

9.1 g. fat
(31% of calories)

1.9 g. dietary fiber

105 mg. cholesterol

631 mg. sodium

PREPARATION TIME
10 minutes

COOKING TIME
25 minutes

PREPARATION TIME
8 minutes

COOKING TIME
50 minutes

French Onion Soup

serves 4

One simple change eliminated a ton of calories and fat from classic onion soup: cooking the onions in a pan coated with no-stick spray rather than sautéing them in a pool of butter and oil.

2   large onions, thinly sliced

4   cups defatted chicken broth

4   cups defatted beef broth

1   clove garlic, minced

1   bay leaf

4   slices French bread or whole-wheat bread, toasted

4   slices mozzarella cheese

Coat a large soup pot with no-stick spray. Place over medium heat and let stand for 1 minute. Add the onions and reduce the heat to low. Cook, stirring often, for 10 minutes, or until the onions are tender.

Add the chicken broth, beef broth, garlic and bay leaf. Cover and bring to a boil. Reduce the heat and simmer for 40 minutes. Remove and discard the bay leaf.

Meanwhile, place the bread on a rack in a broiler pan. Top each slice with mozzarella. Broil about 4" from the heat for 1 minute, or until the cheese is melted. To serve, ladle the soup into bowls and top with the bread.

Hot and Hearty Chowder

serves 4

*This hearty New England soup should hit the spot on really cold evenings.
Serve with a tossed salad and cornbread for a complete meal.*

PER SERVING

252 calories

4.1 g. fat
(15% of calories)

2.5 g. dietary fiber

50 mg. cholesterol

215 mg. sodium

PREPARATION TIME
10 minutes

COOKING TIME
25 minutes

12	shucked chowder clams
5	cups defatted chicken broth
2	large baking potatoes, peeled and diced
1	large onion, diced
1	stalk celery, diced
1	tablespoon minced fresh parsley
1	bay leaf
1/2	teaspoon dried oregano
1/4	teaspoon dried tarragon
1/4	teaspoon ground black pepper
8	ounces cod, cut into 1" pieces
1	cup 1% low-fat milk
1/4	teaspoon black peppercorns

In a large soup pot over medium heat, bring the clams and 2 cups of the broth to a boil. Reduce the heat to medium and simmer for 3 minutes. Remove the clams with a slotted spoon and set aside.

Add the potatoes, onions, celery, parsley, bay leaf, oregano, tarragon, ground pepper and the remaining 3 cups broth to the pot. Bring to a boil. Reduce the heat and simmer for 15 minutes, or until the vegetables are softened. Remove and discard the bay leaf.

Ladle half of the vegetables and 1 cup of the liquid into a blender. Blend until smooth. Return to the pan. Add the cod and simmer for 5 minutes, or until the cod is cooked through.

Chop the clams finely and add to the pan. Stir in the milk and heat briefly. Sprinkle with the peppercorns.

PREPARATION TIME
10 minutes

COOKING TIME
25 minutes

Backyard Garden Tomato Soup

serves 4

Homegrown tomatoes capture the essence of summer in this ripe-red soup. Use the bounty of your own garden or visit a nearby farmers' market for the freshest ingredients. If you hanker after that just-from-the-garden flavor during the winter, canned tomatoes give better flavor than fresh.

1 1/2	cups diced onions
1	sweet red pepper, diced
2	cloves garlic, minced
1	tablespoon olive oil
4	cups chopped plum tomatoes
2	cups water
1/4	cup minced fresh basil
2	tablespoons minced fresh mint

In a large saucepan over medium-high heat, sauté the onions, peppers and garlic in the oil for 1 minute. Cover, reduce the heat to low and cook for 5 minutes.

Add the tomatoes, water, basil and mint. Bring to a boil over medium heat, then reduce the heat and simmer for 15 minutes, or until the vegetables are just tender.

Chef's Note

Mint and tomatoes make a beautiful pair. The sweetness of mint counteracts the natural acidity in tomatoes and eliminates the need for added sugar.

American Harvest Loaf recipe on page 347

PREPARATION TIME
5 minutes

COOKING TIME
20 minutes

Minted Pea Soup

serves 4

This lovely green soup is the essence of spring itself. Use fresh peas when in season and frozen peas the rest of the year.

4	cups water
12	ounces peas
2	cups vegetable broth
1	box (10 ounces) frozen chopped spinach
1	tablespoon chopped fresh mint
1/4	cup 1% low-fat milk
	Salt and ground black pepper

Bring the water to a boil in a large saucepan over high heat. Add the peas and cook for 1 minute. Add the broth, spinach and mint. Reduce the heat and simmer for 20 minutes. Stir in the milk. Add salt and pepper to taste.

Pour the soup into a blender and puree. Serve hot or cold.

Tomato-Orange Soup recipe on page 86

PREPARATION TIME
5 minutes
plus chilling time

COOKING TIME
25 minutes

Photo on page 85

Tomato-Orange Soup

serves 4

Make this refreshing cold soup during the dog days of summer. It comes together quickly and may be made ahead.

1/2	cup chopped onions
1	teaspoon olive oil
1	can (12 ounces) no-salt-added tomatoes, chopped (with juice)
1	tablespoon quick-cooking tapioca
1 1/4	cups vegetable broth
1	cup water
1/4	cup orange juice
1/4	cup 1% low-fat milk
	Salt and ground black pepper

In a large saucepan over medium-high heat, sauté the onions in the oil for 2 minutes, or until soft. Add the tomatoes (with juice), tapioca and ¾ cup of the broth. Reduce the heat and simmer for 20 minutes, or until the soup begins to thicken.

Pour the soup into a blender and puree. Add the water, orange juice, milk and the remaining ½ cup broth. Process to blend. Add salt and pepper to taste. Chill before serving.

Italian Barley Soup

serves 4

Warming and hearty, this soup is typical of Italian home cooking—comforting, effortless and full of good things. It is reliable and sure to please. Serve it with lots of crusty bread and call it a meal.

PER SERVING

318 calories

5.6 g. fat
(15% of calories)

10.3 g. dietary fiber

1 mg. cholesterol

585 mg. sodium

PREPARATION TIME
10 minutes

COOKING TIME
20 minutes

1/2	cup chopped onions
1	teaspoon olive oil
1	ounce prosciutto, diced
1	tablespoon chopped fresh rosemary
1	tablespoon chopped fresh parsley
4	cups defatted chicken broth
1	medium potato, peeled and diced
2	small carrots, diced
1/2	cup quick-cooking barley
2	teaspoons grated Parmesan cheese

In a large saucepan over medium-high heat, sauté the onions in the oil for 3 minutes. Stir in the prosciutto, rosemary and parsley. Cook for 1 minute.

Add the broth, potatoes, carrots and barley. Bring to a boil. Reduce the heat and simmer for 10 to 15 minutes, or until the potatoes are tender. Serve sprinkled with the Parmesan.

Mediterranean Bean and Vegetable Salad Platter

serves 4

This summery dish will remind you of the best antipasto at your favorite Italian restaurant. Our version is low in fat because we've substituted the rich flavor of balsamic vinegar for most of the oil in the dressing.

PREPARATION TIME
10 minutes
plus 20 minutes
marinating time

$1/2$	cup balsamic vinegar
3	tablespoons honey
2	tablespoons minced garlic
2	tablespoons lemon juice
1	tablespoon extra-virgin olive oil
$1/4$	teaspoon salt
2	cups rinsed and drained canned kidney beans
2	cups sliced cooked red potatoes
$1/4$	cup minced red onions
3	cups torn leaf lettuce
$1/2$	cup sliced sweet red peppers
$1/2$	cup sliced green peppers
$1/2$	cup cooked corn
1	large tomato, cut into wedges

In a large bowl, whisk together the vinegar, honey, garlic, lemon juice, oil and salt. Add the beans, potatoes and onions; toss to coat. Let marinate at room temperature for 20 minutes.

Line a platter with the lettuce. Arrange the red peppers, green peppers, corn and tomatoes around the edge. Top with the bean mixture, drizzling the marinade over the vegetables.

PREPARATION TIME
15 minutes

Couscous Salad with Oranges and Olives

serves 4

This zesty salad combines Moroccan influences with Mediterranean ones for a refreshing luncheon dish. You may prepare it several hours ahead and let it come to room temperature before serving.

$3/4$ cup couscous

2 tablespoons frozen orange juice concentrate, thawed

1 tablespoon lemon juice

1 teaspoon Dijon mustard

1 teaspoon extra-virgin olive oil

1 teaspoon chopped fresh oregano

1 teaspoon grated orange rind

1 cup boiling water

1 orange, peeled, sectioned and diced

$1/2$ cup chopped fresh parsley

$1/4$ cup chopped scallions

2 tablespoons sliced black olives

Salt and ground black pepper

In a large bowl, mix the couscous, orange juice concentrate, lemon juice, mustard, oil, oregano and orange rind. Stir in the water. Cover and set aside for 5 minutes, or until the liquid has been absorbed.

Fluff the mixture with a fork. Add the oranges, parsley, scallions and olives; toss to blend. Add salt and pepper to taste.

Chef's Note

Couscous is granular semolina that is sold in the grain and pasta sections of the supermarket. It is ready in just 5 minutes and makes a quick stand-in for pasta and polenta.

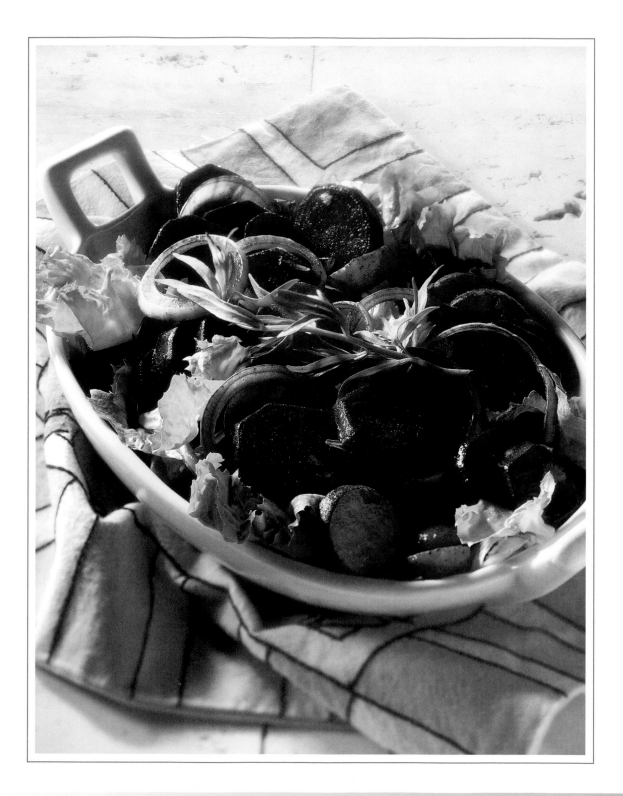

Beet and Potato Salad

serves 4

Magenta beets are especially beautiful in this bright salad served on lovely green escarole.

PER SERVING

131 calories

3.7 g. fat
(24% of calories)

1.1 g. dietary fiber

0 mg. cholesterol

77 mg. sodium

PREPARATION TIME
10 minutes

COOKING TIME
25 minutes

1¼	pounds small beets
8	ounces small red potatoes
2	tablespoons red wine vinegar
1	tablespoon extra-virgin olive oil
2	teaspoons chopped fresh parsley
¾	teaspoon Dijon mustard
¼	teaspoon chopped fresh tarragon
¾	cup thinly sliced onions
	Salt and ground black pepper
4	cups torn escarole

Place the beets and potatoes in separate saucepans. Cover with cold water and bring to a boil over high heat. Reduce the heat to medium and cook until easily pierced with a knife (20 to 25 minutes for the beets and 15 to 20 minutes for the potatoes). Drain and let stand until cool enough to handle. Peel and slice.

In a large bowl, whisk together the vinegar, oil, parsley, mustard and tarragon. Add the beets, potatoes and onions; toss to combine. Add salt and pepper to taste.

Arrange the escarole on a platter. Top with the vegetables and drizzle with the dressing.

PER SERVING

311 calories

4.5 g. fat
(13% of calories)

3.7 g. dietary fiber

37 mg. cholesterol

530 mg. sodium

PREPARATION TIME
10 minutes
plus chilling time

COOKING TIME
10 minutes

Cold Sesame Noodles

serves 4

*A creamy, rich-tasting dressing combines with fast-cooking Japanese udon
noodles to produce an easy cold salad.*

1	pound Japanese udon noodles
1/2	cup fat-free plain yogurt
2	tablespoons reduced-sodium soy sauce
1 1/2	tablespoons honey
1	tablespoon tahini
1	tablespoon peanut butter
1 1/2	cups chopped cooked chicken breast
1	cup julienned carrots
3	scallions, sliced diagonally
1/4	cup chopped fresh parsley

Cook the noodles in a large pot of boiling water according to the package
directions. Drain.

In a large bowl, whisk together the yogurt, soy sauce, honey, tahini and
peanut butter until smooth. Add the chicken, carrots, scallions, parsley and
noodles. Toss to mix well. Chill.

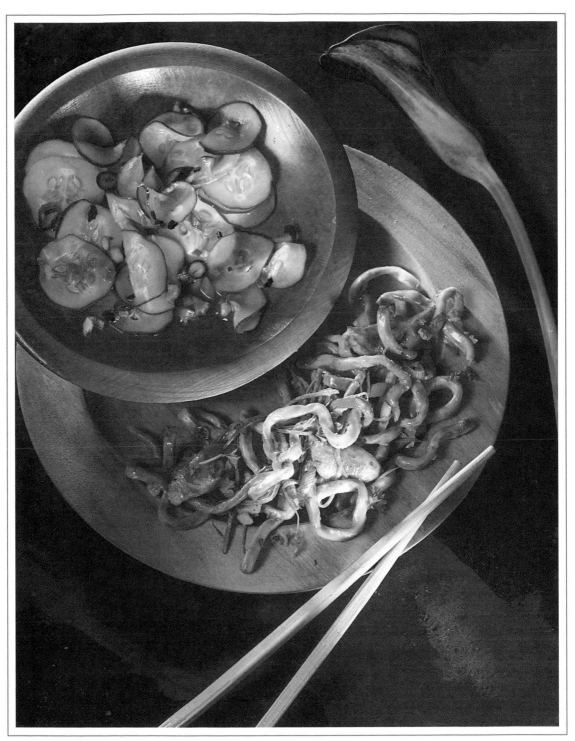

Cucumber Salad recipe on page 115

PER SERVING

388 calories

9.5 g. fat
(22% of calories)

4.5 g. dietary fiber

0 mg. cholesterol

601 mg. sodium

PREPARATION TIME
10 minutes
plus 15 minutes
standing time

Photo on page 71

Panzanella

serves 4

Panzanella is a classic Italian salad containing bread. Serve it in a hollowed-out loaf, as we do here, or over lettuce leaves.

Salad

1	loaf rustic country bread
4	plum tomatoes, chopped
1/4	cup chopped red onions
1/4	cup chopped celery
1/4	cup chopped scallions
1/4	cup chopped fresh basil
1	tablespoon chopped fresh oregano
	Salt and ground black pepper

Dressing

4	teaspoons extra-virgin olive oil
1	tablespoon balsamic vinegar
	Pinch of sugar

TO MAKE THE SALAD
Cut the top off the loaf of bread and pull out all the soft bread inside, leaving a shell. Set the shell aside. Sprinkle the bread pieces and the removed top crust with water and let stand for about 15 minutes, then squeeze out the moisture. Tear the bread into bite-size pieces.

In a large bowl, toss together the bread, tomatoes, onions, celery, scallions, basil and oregano. Add salt and pepper to taste.

TO MAKE THE DRESSING
In a cup, stir together the oil, vinegar and sugar. Pour over the salad and toss to coat.

Serve the salad in the bread shell.

Roasted Eggplant, Pepper and Onion Salad

serves 4

Roasting intensifies the flavors of the vegetables in this colorful salad. It's good served warm or chilled and keeps well for several days in the refrigerator.

PER SERVING

103 calories

3.9 g. fat
(31% of calories)

1.6 g. dietary fiber

0 mg. cholesterol

15 mg. sodium

3	small eggplants, halved lengthwise
2	large sweet red peppers
1	large green pepper
2	small onions, unpeeled and halved
1	tablespoon extra-virgin olive oil
1	tablespoon white wine vinegar
1½	teaspoons balsamic vinegar
1	teaspoon minced garlic
¾	teaspoon drained capers
	Salt and ground black pepper
2	tablespoons chopped fresh parsley

PREPARATION TIME
10 minutes

BAKING TIME
30 minutes

Photo on page 123

Coat a baking sheet with no-stick spray. Place the eggplants, red peppers, green pepper and onions on the sheet. Roast at 400°, turning the vegetables once, for 20 to 30 minutes, or until they are soft and beginning to brown.

Wrap the peppers in damp paper towels and allow to cool for 5 minutes. Peel, halve, remove the seeds and stems and cut the flesh into 1" strips. Cut the eggplants into 1" strips. Peel and dice the onions.

In a large bowl, whisk together the oil, white wine vinegar, balsamic vinegar, garlic and capers. Add the roasted vegetables and toss gently to coat. Add salt and black pepper to taste. Sprinkle with the parsley.

Cobb Salad

serves 4

Cobb salads are as lovely to look at as they are to eat. For maximum effect, arrange the ingredients spoke-fashion on a bed of different varieties of lettuce.

PER SERVING

365 calories

26 g. fat
(65% of calories)

2 g. dietary fiber

170 mg. cholesterol

543 mg. sodium

PREPARATION TIME
15 minutes

1/4	cup extra-virgin olive oil
3	tablespoons white wine vinegar
1/2	teaspoon minced garlic
1/2	teaspoon Worcestershire sauce
2	tablespoons thinly sliced basil leaves
4	cups torn mixed lettuce
8	ounces smoked turkey, cut into strips
2	hard-cooked eggs, chopped
1/2	small red onion, chopped
1	sweet red pepper, chopped
1	yellow pepper, chopped
2	ounces blue cheese, crumbled
1/3	cup diced turkey bacon, cooked until crisp

In a small bowl, whisk together the oil, vinegar, garlic, Worcestershire sauce and basil.

Line a large serving plate with the lettuce. Arrange the turkey, eggs, onions, red peppers and yellow peppers over the lettuce. Sprinkle with the blue cheese and bacon. Drizzle with the dressing.

PREPARATION TIME
25 minutes

Tabbouleh

serves 4

Bulgur is a very fast-cooking grain that's the mainstay of many Middle Eastern salads, including tabbouleh. If you've got red or yellow cherry tomatoes, use them in place of the chopped tomatoes for a prettier presentation.

1	cup defatted chicken broth
1	cup bulgur
2	cups diced tomatoes
$\frac{1}{2}$	cup chopped fresh parsley
$\frac{1}{4}$	cup chopped chives
2	tablespoons chopped fresh mint
3	tablespoons lemon juice
$1\frac{1}{2}$	tablespoons extra-virgin olive oil
1	clove garlic, minced

Bring the broth to a boil in a 1-quart saucepan over high heat. Stir in the bulgur. Cover, remove from the heat and let stand for 15 minutes, or until the bulgur is tender and the liquid has been absorbed. Fluff with a fork and transfer to a large bowl.

Add the tomatoes, parsley, chives and mint. Toss lightly.

In a cup, whisk together the lemon juice, oil and garlic. Pour over the bulgur mixture and toss to mix well.

Southwest Three Bean Salad

serves 4

PER SERVING

204 calories

2.3 g. fat
(9% of calories)

7.4 g. dietary fiber

0 mg. cholesterol

442 mg. sodium

An eye-catching red, white and black, this makes a good luncheon salad or a side dish for grilled chicken or fish, fajitas or burgers. Canned beans work fine; just rinse and drain them to remove excess sodium and packing liquid.

PREPARATION TIME
10 minutes

¼	cup defatted chicken broth
1½	tablespoons red wine vinegar
1	teaspoon extra-virgin olive oil
½	teaspoon chili powder
1	clove garlic, minced
1	cup cooked black beans
1	cup cooked kidney beans
1	cup cooked Great Northern beans
⅓	cup diced red onions
¼	cup diced sweet red peppers
¼	cup minced fresh coriander

In a large bowl, whisk together the broth, vinegar, oil, chili powder and garlic. Add the black beans, kidney beans, Great Northern beans, onions, peppers and coriander. Toss to mix well.

PREPARATION TIME
15 minutes

Wild Rice and Shrimp Salad

serves 4

Wild rice can take up to an hour to cook fully. To make meal preparation quicker, cook the rice ahead of time and refrigerate it until needed.

3	cups cooked wild rice (see note)
12	ounces peeled and deveined shrimp, cooked
1 1/2	cups halved cherry tomatoes
1	can (8 ounces) sliced water chestnuts, drained
1/2	cup cooked peas
1/2	cup sliced scallions
1/2	cup diced red onions
1/4	cup chopped fresh dill
1/4	cup orange juice
1 1/2	tablespoons white wine vinegar
1	tablespoon extra-virgin olive oil
2	teaspoons Dijon mustard
1	clove garlic, minced

In a large bowl, mix the wild rice, shrimp, tomatoes, water chestnuts, peas, scallions, onions and dill.

In a small bowl, whisk together the orange juice, vinegar, oil, mustard and garlic. Drizzle over the salad and toss to combine.

Chef's Note

To cook wild rice: Rinse 1 cup uncooked rice in a strainer until the draining water runs clear. Transfer to a 2-quart saucepan and add 4 cups water and 1 teaspoon salt (optional). Cover and bring to a boil over medium-high heat. Reduce the heat and simmer for 45 to 55 minutes, or until the kernels are open and tender but not mushy. Drain, if necessary. One cup of uncooked wild rice yields 3 to 4 cups cooked.

PREPARATION TIME
15 minutes

COOKING TIME
5 minutes

Roasted Red Pepper Pasta Salad

serves 4

Pureeing roasted red peppers makes a pretty dressing for this light pasta salad. For a heartier dish, add sautéed chicken or turkey breasts.

10	ounces angel hair pasta
4	sweet red peppers, roasted (see note)
¼	cup white wine vinegar
3	tablespoons defatted chicken broth
2	tablespoons chopped fresh parsley
1	tablespoon lemon juice
1	tablespoon extra-virgin olive oil
1	tablespoon chopped fresh oregano
1	teaspoon grated lemon rind
	Salt and ground black pepper

Cook the angel hair in a large pot of boiling water according to the package directions. Drain and transfer to a large bowl.

In a food processor, puree the peppers, vinegar, broth, parsley, lemon juice, oil, oregano and lemon rind; add salt and pepper to taste. Pour over the angel hair and toss to coat. Serve warm or cold.

Chef's Note

To roast peppers, broil about 5" from the heat until charred on all sides. Wrap in damp paper towels and allow to stand for 5 minutes, or until cool enough to handle. Remove and discard the skin, seeds and inner membranes.

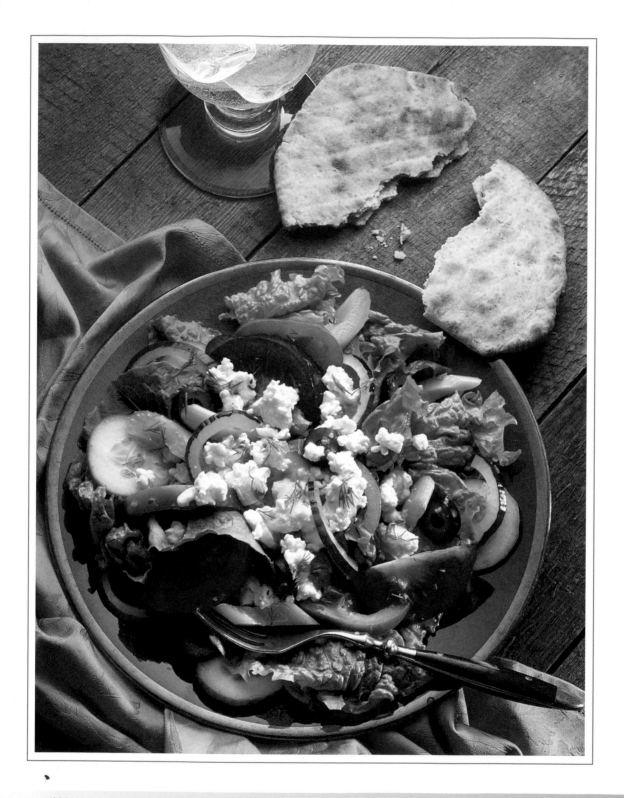

Greek Salata

serves 4

Feta cheese is a hallmark of Greek salads. Here, just a sprinkle of feta gives characteristic flavor without adding a lot of fat.

PER SERVING

92 calories

4.8 g. fat
(47% of calories)

2.7 g. dietary fiber

4 mg. cholesterol

61 mg. sodium

PREPARATION TIME
15 minutes

1	small head red leaf lettuce, torn into bite-size pieces
2	tomatoes, cut into wedges
1	large cucumber, thinly sliced
2	green peppers, sliced
1	small red onion, sliced crosswise and separated into rings
1/3	cup lemon juice
1	tablespoon extra-virgin olive oil
2	teaspoons minced fresh dill
1	clove garlic, minced
2	tablespoons crumbled feta cheese

In a large bowl, toss together the lettuce, tomatoes, cucumbers, peppers, and onions.

In a small bowl, whisk together the lemon juice, oil, dill and garlic. Pour over the tomato mixture and toss to mix well. Serve sprinkled with the feta.

PREPARATION TIME
5 minutes

Black Bean and Corn Salad

serves 4

Here's a Southwestern salad that's perfect for a summer luncheon. To give it more zip, add hot-pepper sauce to taste.

1   cup cooked corn

2   cans (16 ounces each) black beans, rinsed and drained

1/4   cup chopped fresh parsley

2   tablespoons minced red onions

   Salt and ground black pepper

1/4   cup balsamic vinegar

1   tablespoon extra-virgin olive oil

1   teaspoon lemon juice

1   teaspoon minced garlic

1   teaspoon honey or brown sugar

   Lettuce leaves

In a large bowl, mix the corn, beans, parsley and onions. Add salt and pepper to taste.

In a small bowl, whisk together the vinegar, oil, lemon juice, garlic, and honey or brown sugar. Pour over the bean mixture and toss well. Serve over the lettuce.

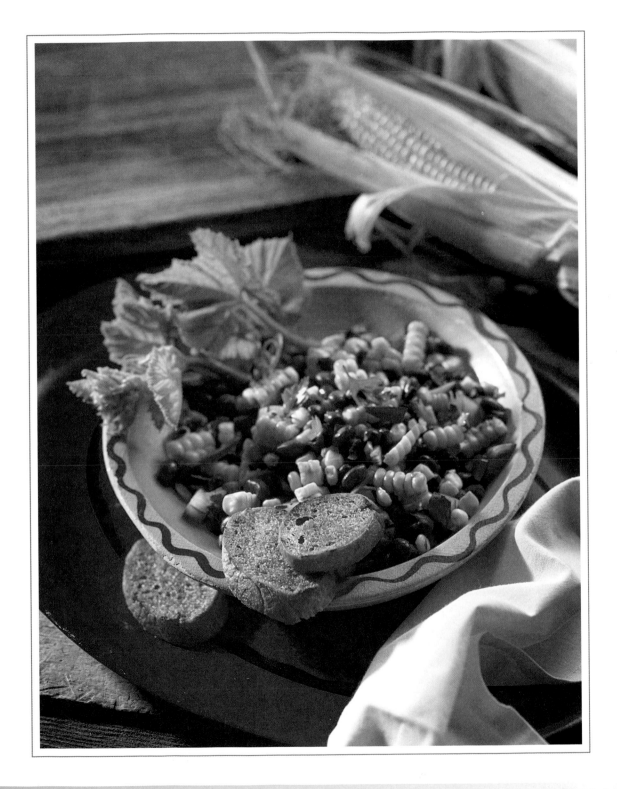

PREPARATION TIME
5 minutes

COOKING TIME
15 minutes

Photo on page 203

Sweet Potato Salad

serves 4

What a delicious way to get disease-fighting beta-carotene! Be sure to choose orange-fleshed sweet potatoes (which are sometimes called yams in supermarkets).

2	large sweet potatoes, peeled and cubed
6	medium red potatoes, cubed
1/2	cup fat-free plain yogurt
1	teaspoon chopped fresh dill
1	tablespoon reduced-fat mayonnaise
1	teaspoon honey mustard
	Salt and ground black pepper
2	tablespoons chopped fresh parsley

Steam the sweet potatoes and red potatoes for about 15 minutes, or until tender.

In a large bowl, whisk together the yogurt, dill, mayonnaise and mustard. Add the potatoes and toss well. Add salt and pepper to taste. Sprinkle with the parsley.

Cucumber Salad

serves 4

Traditional cucumber salads have a high-fat sour cream dressing. This low-fat version is just as refreshing but kinder to your waistline.

PER SERVING

104 calories

1.4 g. fat
(10% of calories)

0.2 g. dietary fiber

0 mg. cholesterol

421 mg. sodium

6	medium cucumbers, peeled, halved lengthwise and thinly sliced
2	tablespoons minced scallions
2	tablespoons brown sugar
$\frac{1}{2}$	cup rice vinegar
3	tablespoons reduced-sodium soy sauce
2	teaspoons finely chopped dry-roasted peanuts
$\frac{1}{4}$	teaspoon red-pepper flakes

In a large bowl, mix the cucumbers, scallions, brown sugar, vinegar and soy sauce. Let marinate for 15 minutes at room temperature.

Add the peanuts and red-pepper flakes. Toss well.

PREPARATION TIME
5 minutes
plus 15 minutes
marinating time

Photo on page 95

chapter 5

Plain and Fancy Poultry

CHICKEN AND TURKEY RULE THE ROOST

The poultry twins—chicken and turkey—have become the mainstay for Americans seeking a healthier diet, and with good reason. They're not only low in fat but also incredibly versatile. Chicken and turkey can be baked, roasted, broiled, grilled, poached, stir-fried and stewed. They're wonderfully suited for all our family favorites, from croquettes and pot pie to stuffed peppers and lasagna. And if that isn't enough, they adapt as well to an elegant after-the-theater dinner party as to an easygoing Saturday-night supper.

PER SERVING

149 calories

3.1 g. fat
(19% of calories)

0 mg. dietary fiber

72 mg. cholesterol

63 mg. sodium

PREPARATION TIME
10 minutes

BAKING TIME
35 minutes

Roasted Chicken
with Lemon and Garlic

serves 4

Great hot or cold, this lemony chicken is perfect for a picnic or a potluck supper. The lemon juice bakes into the chicken so the meat remains moist without additional fat. Leftovers (if there are any) are delicious in salad.

1	fryer chicken (3–3½ pounds)
3	lemons
5	cloves garlic
2	sprigs fresh rosemary

Using a sharp knife, butterfly the chicken by cutting it in half along the top of the breast through the bone. Open the chicken up so that it lies flat and place, cut side down, in a baking pan.

Thinly slice 2 of the lemons. Using your fingers, gently lift the skin up from the breast and work half of the lemon slices under the skin along the breast meat. Tuck the garlic and rosemary under the chicken. Lay the remaining lemon slices on top of the chicken.

Slice the remaining lemon in half. Squeeze the juice of both halves over the chicken.

Roast the chicken at 375° for 10 minutes. Reduce the heat to 350° and continue roasting for 25 minutes, or until the juices run clear when a thigh is tested with a knife. Remove the skin before serving the chicken.

Spicy Corn on the Cob recipe on page 302

Grilled Southwestern-Style Drumsticks

serves 4

Kids will love this one! And since it's about as easy as they come, so will you. Preheat the grill while the chicken marinates.

PER SERVING

204 calories

5.7 g. fat
(25% of calories)

0 g. dietary fiber

82 mg. cholesterol

376 mg. sodium

1	tablespoon garlic powder
1	tablespoon onion powder
1	tablespoon paprika
1	tablespoon chili powder
1	teaspoon ground cumin
1/2	teaspoon salt
1	cup dark beer or apple cider
8	chicken drumsticks, skin removed

PREPARATION TIME
5 minutes
plus 20 minutes
marinating time

COOKING TIME
20 minutes

In a resealable plastic bag, combine the garlic powder, onion powder, paprika, chili powder, cumin, and salt. Shake the bag to mix. Add the beer or apple cider and drumsticks. Shake well. Refrigerate for 20 minutes or up to 24 hours, turning occasionally.

Remove the drumsticks from the bag; reserve the marinade. Place the drumsticks on a plate and lightly coat with no-stick spray.

Grill for 20 minutes, or until the juices run clear when a drumstick is tested with a knife. Baste occasionally during the first 15 minutes with the reserved marinade. Discard the remaining marinade.

PREPARATION TIME
5 minutes

COOKING TIME
20 minutes

Lemon-Herb Chicken Breasts

serves 4

Serve this lemony chicken over pasta, rice or polenta to soak up the herb-infused juices.

2	tablespoons all-purpose flour
	Salt and ground black pepper
4	boneless, skinless chicken breasts halves (4 ounces each)
1	clove garlic, minced
¼	cup defatted chicken broth
12	thin strips lemon rind
2	tablespoons lemon juice
1	teaspoon chopped fresh oregano
1	tablespoon chopped fresh basil

Season the flour with salt and pepper to taste. Dip the chicken in the flour to coat lightly on all sides; shake off excess flour.

In a large no-stick frying pan over medium-high heat, sauté the garlic for 1 minute, or until soft. Add the chicken and sauté for 5 minutes per side, or until cooked through and no longer pink when cut with a knife. Transfer the chicken to a plate.

Add the broth, lemon rind, lemon juice, and oregano to the pan and bring to a boil. Reduce the heat and simmer for 5 minutes, or until the liquid is reduced by half. Return the chicken to the pan to warm through. Sprinkle with the basil.

Roasted Eggplant, Pepper and Onion Salad recipe on page 97

PREPARATION TIME
10 minutes

COOKING TIME
25 minutes

Chicken Cacciatore

serves 4

Cacciatore means "hunter," and this chicken dish, made with dark-meat thighs, is reminiscent of the game dishes of the Italian countryside: fragrant stews of tomatoes, onions and herbs. Serve this over rice to absorb the sauce.

4	chicken thighs (5 ounces each)
2	cups chopped canned tomatoes, drained
1	cup chopped mushrooms
¼	cup red wine or defatted chicken broth
¼	cup chopped fresh parsley
3	cloves garlic, minced
4	black olives, pitted and chopped
2	cups hot cooked brown rice

Remove the skin and any excess fat from the chicken.

Coat a large no-stick frying pan with no-stick spray. Place over medium heat until hot. Add the chicken and brown on all sides.

Add the tomatoes, mushrooms, wine or broth, parsley and garlic. Reduce the heat and simmer for 20 minutes, or until the chicken is tender and no longer pink when tested with a knife.

Stir in the olives. Serve over the rice.

Chef's Note

Use a combination of different mushrooms for the most flavor.
Good choices include portobello, shiitake, cremini and button mushrooms.

Turkey Noodle Casserole

serves 4

This old-fashioned casserole has been updated and streamlined with cooked turkey and a low-fat cheese sauce. Serve with steamed broccoli and baked potatoes to round out a classic dinner.

PER SERVING

617 calories

12.6 g. fat
(18% of calories)

3.3 g. dietary fiber

129 mg. cholesterol

642 mg. sodium

PREPARATION TIME
20 minutes

BAKING TIME
30 minutes

4	cups sliced mushrooms
1	tablespoon water
2	teaspoons olive oil
1/3	cup minced onions
2	tablespoons white wine or apple juice
1/4	cup all-purpose flour
2	cups defatted chicken broth
1 3/4	cups skim milk
1/4	cup reduced-fat cream cheese
1/2	teaspoon dried thyme
10	ounces yolk-free noodles
2	cups chopped cooked turkey breast
1	cup frozen peas
1	jar (2 ounces) diced pimientos
1/3	cup grated Parmesan cheese
1/3	cup seasoned bread crumbs
1/2	teaspoon ground black pepper

In a 2-quart saucepan, mix the mushrooms, water and oil. Cook over medium-high heat, stirring frequently, for 7 minutes, or until the mushrooms brown and the pan is dry. Add the onions and wine or apple juice. Cook for 2 minutes.

Stir in the flour and cook for 3 minutes. Gradually stir in the broth, milk, cream cheese and thyme. Cook, stirring, for 5 minutes, or until the sauce has slightly thickened.

Cook the noodles in a large pot of boiling water according to the package directions. Drain well and transfer to a large bowl. Stir in the mushroom sauce, turkey, peas, pimientos and Parmesan.

Coat a 3-quart casserole with no-stick spray. Add the turkey mixture. Sprinkle with the bread crumbs and pepper. Bake at 375° for 20 to 30 minutes, or until bubbling.

Plain and Fancy Poultry

Mediterranean Turkey
in Apricot Sauce

serves 4

The apricots and pine nuts in this sweet and tart sauce give seared turkey breast exotic flavor.

PER SERVING

334 calories

3.4 g. fat
(9% of calories)

2.4 g. dietary fiber

74 mg. cholesterol

170 mg. sodium

PREPARATION TIME
5 minutes

COOKING TIME
20 minutes

4	turkey breast slices (4 ounces each)
1	cup defatted chicken broth
1	cup orange juice
1/4	cup coarsely chopped dried apricots
1	tablespoon white wine vinegar
1	teaspoon honey
2	cups hot cooked rice
2	tablespoons toasted pine nuts

In a large no-stick frying pan over medium-high heat, sear the turkey for 2 minutes per side. Transfer to a plate.

Add the broth, orange juice, apricots, vinegar and honey to the pan. Simmer for 10 minutes, or until the liquid is reduced by half.

Return the turkey to the pan and simmer for 2 to 3 minutes, or until the meat is no longer pink when tested with a knife. Serve over the rice and sprinkle with the pine nuts.

Chicken Parmesan

serves 4

Breaded cutlets are an American tradition. To trim the fat from this popular recipe, we used just a smidgen of olive oil and baked the cutlets rather than pan-frying them. This dish is delicious served on a bed of hot pasta.

1	tablespoon olive oil
1	tablespoon minced garlic
$1/2$	teaspoon ground black pepper
2	teaspoons dried oregano
1	cup fresh bread crumbs
2	tablespoons grated Parmesan cheese
4	boneless, skinless chicken breast halves (4 ounces each)
1	cup tomato sauce, heated

In a shallow bowl, mix the oil, garlic, pepper and 1 teaspoon of the oregano. On a sheet of wax paper, mix the bread crumbs, Parmesan and the remaining 1 teaspoon oregano.

Dip the chicken into the oil mixture to coat both sides. Dip into the bread crumb mixture to coat well.

Coat a baking sheet with no-stick spray. Place the chicken on the sheet and mist with no-stick spray. Bake at 400° for 5 minutes. Turn the pieces and bake for 10 minutes, or until the chicken is crisp and golden brown.

Serve topped with the tomato sauce.

PER SERVING

158 calories

4.6 g. fat
(27% of calories)

0.7 g. dietary fiber

48 mg. cholesterol

260 mg. sodium

PREPARATION TIME
10 minutes

BAKING TIME
15 minutes

PREPARATION TIME
10 minutes
plus 15 minutes
marinating time

COOKING TIME
10 minutes

Florida Chicken

serves 4

Florida's cuisine blends locally grown citrus fruit with the fire-and-spice seasonings imported from the Caribbean. For a special dinner, serve this chicken in a hollowed-out pineapple half.

Chicken and Marinade

2	tangerines
1/4	cup pineapple juice
1/8	teaspoon ground allspice
1/8	teaspoon ground mace
1/8	teaspoon ground ginger
1/8	teaspoon ground red pepper
4	boneless, skinless chicken breast halves (4 ounces each)

Fruit Sauce

1	cup orange sections
1/2	cup pineapple cubes
1/2	cup sliced strawberries
1	tablespoon chopped fresh mint

TO MAKE THE CHICKEN AND MARINADE

Cut the tangerines in half crosswise and remove the seeds. Chop the rind and flesh coarsely and place in a food processor. Add the pineapple juice, allspice, mace, ginger and pepper. Process for 20 seconds, or until pureed. Reserve 1 tablespoon of the marinade and place in a medium bowl; set aside.

Pour the remaining marinade into a shallow bowl and add the chicken. Turn the pieces to coat all over. Cover and marinate for 15 minutes in the refrigerator.

Remove the chicken from the marinade; discard the marinade. Broil or grill the chicken for 4 to 5 minutes per side, or until cooked through and no longer pink when tested with a knife.

TO MAKE THE FRUIT SAUCE

Add the oranges, pineapple, strawberries and mint to the bowl containing the 1 tablespoon reserved marinade. Mix well and serve with the chicken.

Chef's Note

Clementines, minneolas and navel oranges are all suitable replacements for the tangerines.

PREPARATION TIME
5 minutes

COOKING TIME
10 minutes

Grilled Chicken Sandwiches with Sun-Dried Tomato Mayonnaise

serves 4

Sun-drying makes tomatoes chewy, deep red and intensely flavorful.

1/4	cup reduced-fat mayonnaise
4	cloves garlic, roasted (see note)
2	tablespoons minced sun-dried tomatoes packed in oil
1	teaspoon lemon juice
1/2	teaspoon Dijon mustard
4	boneless, skinless chicken breast halves (4 ounces each)
4	thick slices sourdough bread

In a small bowl, mix the mayonnaise, garlic, tomatoes, lemon juice and mustard.

Grill the chicken for 3 to 4 minutes per side, or until cooked through and no longer pink when tested with a knife.

Coat both sides of the bread with no-stick spray. Grill for 1 minute per side. Spread 1 tablespoon of the mayonnaise mixture on each slice and top with the chicken.

Chef's Note

Roasting mellows and sweetens garlic. To roast garlic, place unpeeled cloves on a piece of aluminum foil, coat with no-stick spray and add 1 teaspoon water. Seal the foil. Bake at 400° until the garlic softens, about 15 minutes. Squeeze the cloves from their skin.

Tahini Chicken

serves 4

A spicy tahini sauce helps dress up leftover cooked chicken. Serve the chicken over rice or couscous.

PER SERVING

205 calories

10 g. fat
(43% of calories)

1.3 g. dietary fiber

48 mg. cholesterol

512 mg. sodium

³⁄₄	cup defatted chicken broth
¹⁄₄	cup tahini
2	tablespoons reduced-sodium soy sauce
1	tablespoon honey
1	clove garlic, minced
2	teaspoons grated fresh ginger
1	teaspoon hot-pepper sauce
2	cups cubed cooked chicken breast

PREPARATION TIME
10 minutes

COOKING TIME
5 minutes

Bring the broth to a boil in a 2-quart saucepan over medium heat. Reduce the heat to low. Whisk in the tahini, soy sauce, honey, garlic, ginger and hot-pepper sauce until smooth. Stir in the chicken. Heat through.

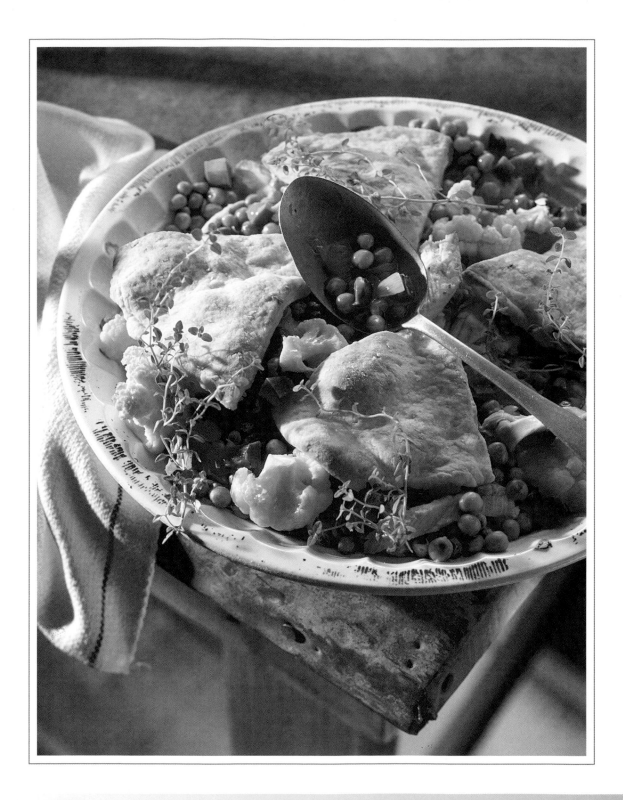

Plain and Fancy Poultry

Turkey Pot Pie
with Buttermilk Biscuit Crust

serves 4

Yes! You can have old-fashioned turkey pot pie in less than 45 minutes. Cooked turkey and frozen mixed vegetables help streamline this family favorite.

1	cup all-purpose flour
1	teaspoon baking powder
1/4	teaspoon baking soda
	Pinch of salt
1	tablespoon plus 2 teaspoons chilled butter, cut into small pieces
1/4	cup low-fat buttermilk
3	tablespoons reduced-fat sour cream
1 3/4	cups defatted chicken broth
1/3	cup chopped onions
2	teaspoons minced garlic
2 1/2	tablespoons cornstarch
1/4	teaspoon poultry seasoning
1/2	teaspoon dried thyme
1/4	teaspoon dried sage
2	cups frozen mixed peas, carrots and cauliflower, thawed
2	cups diced cooked turkey breast

In a medium bowl, mix the flour, baking powder, baking soda and salt. Cut in the butter with 2 knives until the mixture resembles fine crumbs. Stir in the buttermilk and sour cream to form a dough. Turn the dough onto a sheet of plastic wrap and flatten it into a large disk; wrap tightly. Refrigerate while you make the filling.

Bring 1/4 cup of the broth to a boil in a large frying pan. Add the onions and garlic. Cook for 2 minutes.

In a small bowl, mix the cornstarch, poultry seasoning, thyme, and sage. Stir in the remaining 1 1/2 cups broth until smooth. Add to the frying pan. Cook until the mixture comes to a boil and thickens. Remove from the heat and add the vegetables and turkey. Pour into an 8" × 8" baking dish.

Cut the biscuit dough into four sections; arrange on top of the filling. Bake at 425° for 30 minutes, or until the biscuits are golden brown and the filling is bubbling.

PER SERVING

331 calories

6.4 g. fat
(18% of calories)

3.2 g. dietary fiber

64 mg. cholesterol

536 mg. sodium

PREPARATION TIME
15 minutes

BAKING TIME
30 minutes

PREPARATION TIME
10 minutes

COOKING TIME
30 minutes

Chicken and Seafood Gumbo

serves 6

Filé powder (ground sassafras leaves) is what gives gumbo authentic Creole flavor. Look for it in the spice section of the supermarket.

1	tablespoon canola oil
1	tablespoon all-purpose flour
1½	cups diced onions
1	green pepper, diced
¼	cup diced celery
1	can (14½ ounces) no-salt-added tomatoes, chopped
1	can (10 ounces) tomatoes with chilies, chopped
1½	cups water
8	ounces boneless, skinless chicken breast, diced
8	ounces peeled and deveined shrimp
1	cup shucked oysters
½	teaspoon filé powder
2	cups hot cooked rice

In a 4-quart saucepan, mix the oil and flour. Cook, stirring constantly, over medium heat for 3 to 5 minutes, or until the mixture turns dark brown but does not burn. Add the onions, peppers and celery. Cook for 3 to 4 minutes, or until the vegetables begin to soften.

Add the tomatoes, tomatoes with chilies and water; bring to a boil. Cook for 10 minutes. Add the chicken and cook for 5 minutes. Add the shrimp, oysters and filé powder and cook for 5 minutes, or just until the seafood is cooked through. Serve with the rice.

Plain and Fancy Poultry

Chicken Casserole
with Herbed Lemon Biscuits

serves 4

Cake flour added to these biscuits keeps them light and fluffy.

PER SERVING

479 calories

22.4 g. fat
(42% of calories)

3.6 g. dietary fiber

72 mg. cholesterol

458 mg. sodium

Herbed Lemon Biscuits

½	cup all-purpose flour
¼	cup whole-wheat flour
¼	cup cake flour
2	teaspoons baking powder
1	teaspoon dried dill
¼	teaspoon salt
½	cup low-fat buttermilk
¼	cup canola oil
1	teaspoon grated lemon rind

Chicken Casserole

½	cup pearl onions
2	teaspoons canola oil
12	ounces boneless, skinless chicken breast, cut into ½" pieces
1	cup diced cooked potatoes
1	cup snow peas
½	cup thinly sliced cooked carrots
½	cup defatted chicken broth
¼	teaspoon dried tarragon
¼	teaspoon ground black pepper
¼	teaspoon dried dill
2	teaspoons cornstarch
1	tablespoon cold water

PREPARATION TIME
15 minutes

COOKING TIME
15 minutes

BAKING TIME
15 minutes

TO MAKE THE HERBED LEMON BISCUITS

In a medium bowl, mix the all-purpose flour, whole-wheat flour, cake flour, baking powder, dill and salt.

In a small bowl, mix the buttermilk, oil and lemon rind. Add to the flour mixture and stir until moistened.

(continued)

Coat a baking sheet with no-stick spray. Drop 6 mounds of the dough onto the sheet. Bake at 425° for 15 minutes, or until golden.

TO MAKE THE CHICKEN CASSEROLE

In a 2-quart saucepan over medium heat, sauté the onions in the oil for 6 minutes, or until golden brown. Add the chicken and stir for 3 minutes. Add the potatoes, snow peas, carrots, broth, tarragon, pepper and dill. Cook over medium-low heat until the mixture boils.

In a cup, mix the cornstarch and water until smooth. Stir into the saucepan. Cook for 2 minutes, or until the mixture thickens. Transfer to a serving dish. Top with the biscuits.

Turkey Stir-Fry

serves 4

PER SERVING

250 calories

5.5 g. fat
(20% of calories)

2.1 g. dietary fiber

79 mg. cholesterol

288 mg. sodium

You may vary the vegetables to accommodate what's on hand. Serve the stir-fry over rice.

1	tablespoon minced fresh ginger
1	clove garlic, minced
1	tablespoon apricot preserves
1	tablespoon reduced-sodium soy sauce
1	tablespoon white vinegar
1	pound boneless, skinless turkey breast
1	large onion, thinly sliced
4	ounces snow peas
1	sweet red pepper, thinly sliced
2	teaspoons canola oil
1	tablespoon cornstarch
¾	cup defatted chicken broth

PREPARATION TIME
15 minutes

COOKING TIME
15 minutes

In a large bowl, mix the ginger, garlic, preserves, soy sauce and vinegar. Cut the turkey into thin strips, add to the bowl and mix well.

In a large no-stick frying pan over medium-high heat, stir-fry the onions, snow peas and peppers in the oil for 5 minutes, or until just tender. Remove with a slotted spoon and set aside.

Add the turkey, with the marinade, to the pan. Stir-fry for 5 minutes, or until the turkey is cooked through. Return the vegetables to the pan.

In a cup, mix the cornstarch and broth until smooth. Add to the pan. Stir until thick.

PREPARATION TIME
5 minutes
plus 15 minutes
marinating time

COOKING TIME
25 minutes

Grilled Raspberry Turkey Breasts

serves 4

Raspberry sauce makes this turkey taste rich and satisfying—without any added fat. You can let the turkey marinate all day so it's ready to grill when you get home from work.

1	cup raspberry vinegar
1/2	cup frozen unsweetened raspberries
2	cloves garlic, minced
2	teaspoons minced fresh ginger
1	tablespoon reduced-sodium soy sauce
1	boneless, skinless turkey breast half (1 pound)

In a resealable plastic bag, combine the vinegar, raspberries, garlic, ginger and soy sauce. Add the turkey and shake well. Refrigerate for 15 minutes or up to 24 hours, turning occasionally.

Remove the turkey from the bag and wrap in a piece of aluminum foil (reserve the marinade). Grill for 20 minutes.

Strain the marinade into a small saucepan by pressing it through a strainer with rubber spatula. Cook over high heat until reduced to 1/3 cup.

Unwrap the turkey and place it directly on the grill. Cook for 5 minutes, or until the turkey is cooked through and no longer pink when tested with a knife; turn once and baste with the reduced marinade during this time. Transfer to a serving platter and top with the remaining reduced marinade.

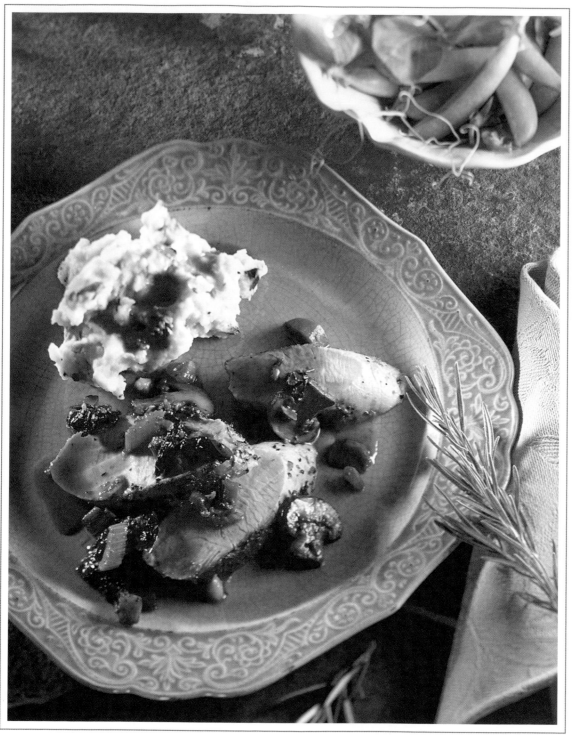

Garlic Mashed Potatoes recipe on page 294

Turkey Tenderloin with Tomato-Mushroom Sauce

serves 4

PER SERVING

203 calories

4 g. fat
(17% of calories)

2.8 g. dietary fiber

44 mg. cholesterol

201 mg. sodium

Garlic-flavored mashed potatoes would be an ideal accompaniment to this easy entrée.

1	pound turkey tenderloin, cut into 4 pieces
2	tablespoons seasoned bread crumbs
1	teaspoon olive oil
1/4	cup defatted chicken broth
1/2	cup chopped onions
1	teaspoon minced garlic
1/2	cup diced carrots
1/2	cup diced celery
1	cup sliced mushrooms
2	ounces dry-pack sun-dried tomatoes, chopped
1	cup chopped tomatoes
1/4	teaspoon dried rosemary
	Salt and ground black pepper

PREPARATION TIME
10 minutes

COOKING TIME
30 minutes

Place the turkey and bread crumbs in a resealable plastic bag; shake well.

Warm the oil in a large no-stick frying pan over medium-high heat. Add the turkey. Cook for 2 minutes on each side. Transfer to a plate.

Add the broth, onions, garlic, carrots, celery, mushrooms, sun-dried tomatoes, chopped tomatoes and rosemary to the frying pan. Cook for 5 minutes. Add the turkey. Cover and reduce the heat to medium. Cook for 20 minutes, or until the turkey is cooked through and no longer pink when tested with a knife.

PREPARATION TIME
10 minutes

BAKING TIME
30 minutes

Chicken and
Black Bean Lasagna

serves 4

Bake two pans of this zesty lasagna at a time—one to enjoy now, the other to freeze for later. To easily freeze lasagna, line the baking dish with foil before assembling the lasagna; freeze uncovered. When frozen, remove the lasagna from the dish, wrap in the foil and return to the freezer.

1	can (28 ounces) low-sodium tomatoes, drained and chopped
1	can (4 ounces) chopped green chili peppers, drained
1	can (8 ounces) low-sodium tomato sauce
1	can (15 ounces) black beans, rinsed and drained
1	teaspoon ground cumin
1	teaspoon chili powder
6	no-boil lasagna noodles
1½	cups fat-free ricotta cheese
2	cups chopped cooked chicken breast
2	cups shredded reduced-fat Cheddar cheese

In a medium bowl, mix the tomatoes, peppers and tomato sauce.

In a small bowl, mix the beans, cumin and chili powder. Lightly mash the beans with a fork.

Coat an 8" × 8" baking dish with no-stick spray. Spoon ½ cup of the tomato mixture into the dish.

Place 2 of the noodles over the sauce. Top with one-third of the beans, one-third of the ricotta and one-third of the chicken. Cover with ½ cup of the Cheddar and one-third of the remaining tomato sauce. Repeat twice.

Top with the remaining ½ cup Cheddar.

Bake at 375° for 30 minutes, or until bubbling.

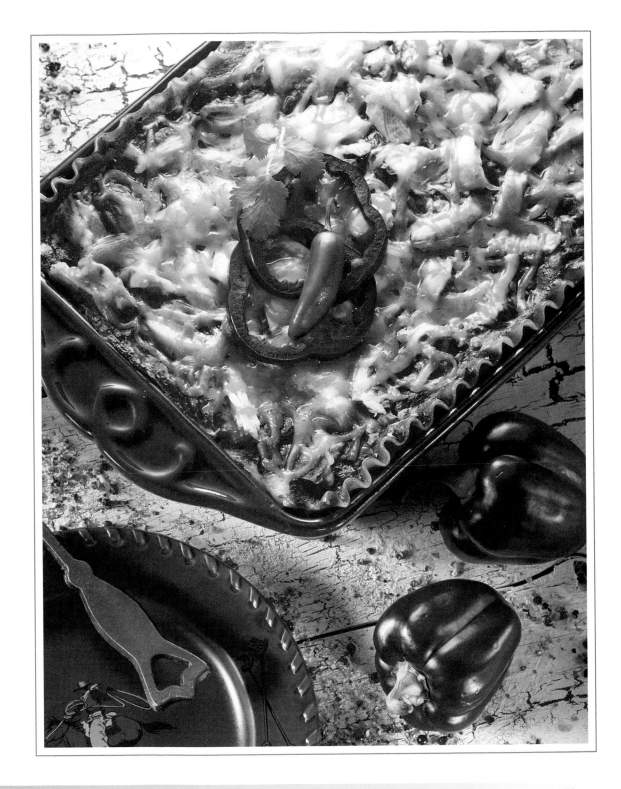

PER SERVING

356 calories

6.5 g. fat
(16% of calories)

9.9 g. dietary fiber

26 mg. cholesterol

810 mg. sodium

PREPARATION TIME
20 minutes

BAKING TIME
30 minutes

Quick Cassoulet

serves 4

Cassoulet is a classic French bean and meat casserole that generally takes a long time to prepare. You can make it much faster by using canned beans. What's more, you can turn out a considerably leaner version by replacing the traditional pork, lamb, duck and regular sausage with smoked turkey breast and turkey sausage.

6	ounces mild or spicy turkey sausage links
1	large onion, diced
1	tart apple, diced
1	cup defatted chicken broth
2	tablespoons tomato paste
2	cans (19 ounces each) navy beans, rinsed and drained
3	ounces smoked turkey breast, diced
$^1/_2$	teaspoon dried thyme
$^1/_2$	teaspoon ground black pepper
1	cup fresh bread crumbs
$^1/_2$	cup minced fresh parsley
2	teaspoons olive oil

Brown the sausage in a large no-stick frying pan over medium heat. Transfer to a cutting board and slice into $^1/_2$" pieces. Return to the pan and add the onions, apples and 2 tablespoons of the broth. Sauté for 5 minutes, or until the onions and apples are softened. Stir in the tomato paste and the remaining broth.

Transfer to a large bowl. Stir in the beans, turkey breast, thyme and pepper.

Coat a 3-quart casserole with no-stick spray. Add the bean mixture.

In a small bowl, mix the bread crumbs, parsley and oil. Sprinkle over the bean mixture. Bake at 350° for 30 minutes.

Chef's Note

To make fresh bread crumbs, tear bread slices into large chunks. Place in a food processor and grind with on/off turns. You may use any type of bread, including whole-wheat, oat, multigrain or white.

Turkey Parmesan

serves 4

PER SERVING

297 calories

5.7 g. fat
(17% of calories)

1 g. dietary fiber

71 mg. cholesterol

550 mg. sodium

Old-fashioned recipes for Parmesan cutlets call for frying the pieces in lots of oil. Here, we bake the cutlets to keep them lean.

PREPARATION TIME
10 minutes

BAKING TIME
10 minutes

2	tablespoons all-purpose flour
1/4	teaspoon ground black pepper
1/2	cup fat-free egg substitute
3/4	cup dry bread crumbs
1/4	cup grated Parmesan cheese
1	pound turkey breast cutlets, about 1/4" thick
1	cup tomato sauce, heated

Combine the flour and pepper on a sheet of wax paper. Place the egg substitute in a shallow bowl. Combine the bread crumbs and Parmesan on another sheet of wax paper.

Dip the turkey into the flour mixture to lightly coat both sides. Dip each cutlet first into the egg substitute and then into the Parmesan mixture to coat well.

Coat a large baking sheet with no-stick spray. Place the cutlets on the sheet. Bake at 400° for 5 minutes. Turn the pieces and bake for 5 minutes, or until the cutlets are golden and crisp. Serve topped with the tomato sauce.

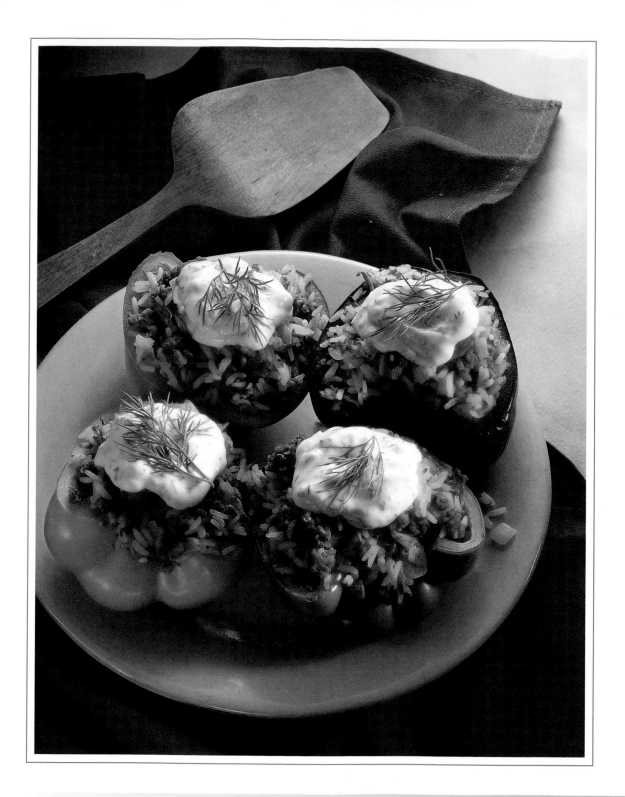

Plain and Fancy Poultry

Turkey Stuffed Peppers

serves 4

Red and green peppers are the serving "boats" for well-seasoned turkey-rice stuffing in this recipe. For variety, try other colors of peppers such as yellow and purple, but remember that purple peppers turn green when cooked.

PREPARATION TIME
20 minutes

BAKING TIME
15 minutes

1	large sweet red pepper
1	large green pepper
1½	cups cooked brown rice
½	cup diced onions
¼	cup defatted chicken broth
1	teaspoon grated orange rind
½	teaspoon ground black pepper
6	ounces ground turkey breast
1	carrot, shredded
¼	cup diced dill pickles
1	egg white
3	cloves garlic
1	teaspoon Dijon mustard
¼	cup fat-free sour cream
½	teaspoon dried dill

Cut the peppers in half lengthwise and remove the seeds and membranes. Place in a pot of boiling water for 1 minute. Drain.

In a large no-stick frying pan, mix the rice, onions, broth, orange rind and black pepper. Cook over medium heat for 3 minutes. Add the turkey and cook, breaking up the pieces with a spoon, until the turkey is no longer pink. Remove from the heat.

Stir in the carrots, pickles, egg white, garlic and mustard.

Fill the pepper halves with the turkey mixture. Place in a shallow pan large enough to hold the pepper halves in a single layer. Pour about ½" of water into the pan and bake at 375° for 15 minutes.

In a cup, mix the sour cream and dill. Serve with the peppers.

PREPARATION TIME
5 minutes

COOKING TIME
25 minutes

Milan-Style Turkey Stew

serves 4

This light, lemony stew was inspired by osso buco, a Milanese dish that slow-cooks vegetables and veal shanks until meltingly tender. It is traditionally served with gremolada, an aromatic mixture of lemon rind, garlic and parsley.

$^1/_2$	cup finely chopped onions
$^1/_2$	cup finely chopped carrots
$^1/_2$	cup finely chopped celery
1	tablespoon grated lemon rind
1	clove garlic, minced
1	pound boneless, skinless turkey thighs, cut into 2" cubes
1	can (14$^1/_2$ ounces) no-salt-added tomatoes, chopped (with juice)
1	cup white wine or defatted chicken broth
2	tablespoons lemon juice
1	teaspoon dried oregano
3	sprigs fresh parsley
1	bay leaf
	Salt and ground black pepper
	Gremolada (see note)

In a large no-stick frying pan over medium heat, cook the onions, carrots, celery, lemon rind and garlic for 2 minutes, or until soft. Add the turkey and continue to cook, stirring constantly, for 2 minutes, or until the turkey begins to brown.

Add the tomatoes (with juice), wine or broth, lemon juice, oregano, parsley and bay leaf. Cover, reduce the heat and cook for 5 minutes. Uncover and simmer for 15 minutes, or until the sauce thickens.

Add salt and pepper to taste. Remove and discard the parsley and bay leaf. Serve sprinkled with the gremolada.

Chef's Note

To make gremolada: Mix 1 tablespoon finely chopped fresh parsley, 1 teaspoon grated lemon rind and $^1/_2$ teaspoon minced garlic.

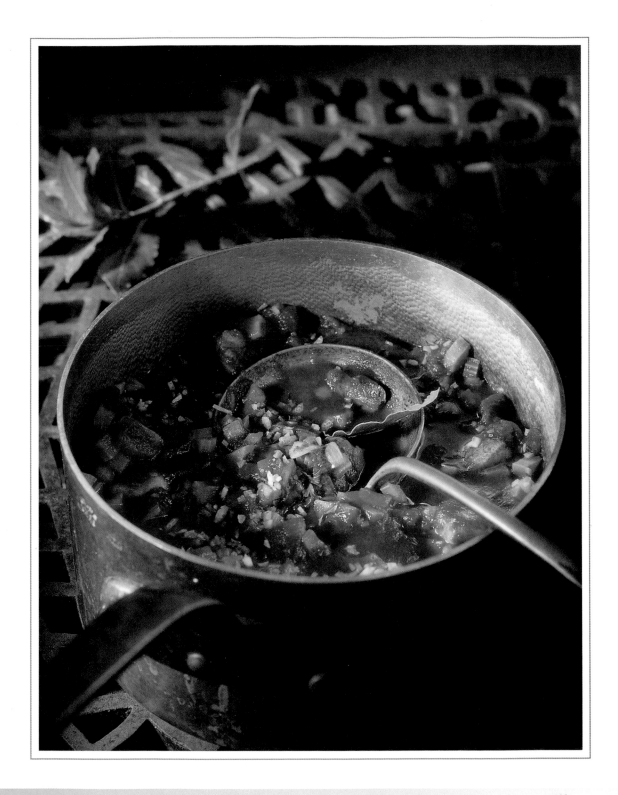

PREPARATION TIME
15 minutes
plus 15 minutes
chilling time

COOKING TIME
10 minutes

Turkey Croquettes

serves 4

Here's a time-honored way to use up leftover cooked turkey. But unlike traditional croquettes, these are lightly sautéed, not deep-fried.

4	cups diced cooked turkey
1/2	cup diced onions
1/4	cup diced celery
1/4	cup minced fresh parsley
2	hard-cooked egg whites, finely chopped
1/3	cup fat-free mayonnaise
2	teaspoons Worcestershire sauce
1/2	teaspoon paprika
1/4	teaspoon dry mustard
1/4	teaspoon ground black pepper
1	egg white
1 1/2	cups fresh bread crumbs
1	teaspoon olive oil
1 1/2	cups fat-free plain yogurt
2	tablespoons chopped chives
1	teaspoon lemon juice

In a large bowl, mix the turkey, onions, celery, parsley and cooked egg whites.

In a small bowl, whisk together the mayonnaise, Worcestershire sauce, paprika, mustard and pepper. Stir into the turkey mixture and blend well. Form into 4 thick patties. Cover and refrigerate for at least 15 minutes to set the mixture.

Place the egg white in a shallow bowl and beat lightly with a fork. Place the bread crumbs on a sheet of wax paper. Dip each patty first into the egg white, then into the bread crumbs to coat well.

Warm the oil in a large no-stick frying pan over medium-high heat. Add the patties and sauté for 5 minutes per side, or until golden.

In a small bowl, whisk together the yogurt, chives and lemon juice. Serve as a sauce with the patties.

Lemon Turkey Tenders

serves 4

Turkey tenders are cutlets from the breast. To garnish this lemon chicken–like recipe, roll peeled lemon slices in fresh minced herbs such as thyme or mint. Place a lemon slice on each plate or arrange them on the serving platter.

PER SERVING

186 calories

5.3 g. fat
(26% of calories)

1 g. dietary fiber

71 mg. cholesterol

104 mg. sodium.

PREPARATION TIME
10 minutes

COOKING TIME
10 minutes

4	turkey breast cutlets, ¼" thick
¼	cup whole-wheat flour
4	teaspoons canola oil
1	teaspoon cornstarch
1	tablespoon cold water
½	cup defatted chicken broth
1	teaspoon grated lemon rind
1	teaspoon chopped fresh thyme

Dredge the cutlets in the flour. Heat the oil in a large no-stick skillet. Add the cutlets and cook for 1 minute per side, or until a light golden brown. Remove the turkey from the pan.

In a cup, mix the cornstarch and water.

Add the broth, lemon rind, and thyme to the pan. Bring to a boil. Add the cornstarch mixture to the pan. Cook over medium heat for 2 minutes, or until the mixture thickens and becomes glossy. Add the turkey. Heat for 2 minutes and serve.

chapter 6

Seafood for All Occasions

FAMILY PLEASERS PLUS COMPANY FARE

Littleneck clams, rainbow trout and walleyed pike. Catfish, soft-shelled crabs and shrimp. Lobster, salmon and orange roughy. This list just begins to touch on the incredible variety of finned and shelled creatures that inhabit our lakes, rivers and oceans—and lend versatility and flavor to our diets. Seafood and fish—often called "brain food," and for good reason—are excellent sources of a whole alphabet of vitamins and minerals from vitamin A to zinc. Many fish are virtually fat-free, and what fat they do contain is in the form of heart-healthy omega-3 fatty acids.

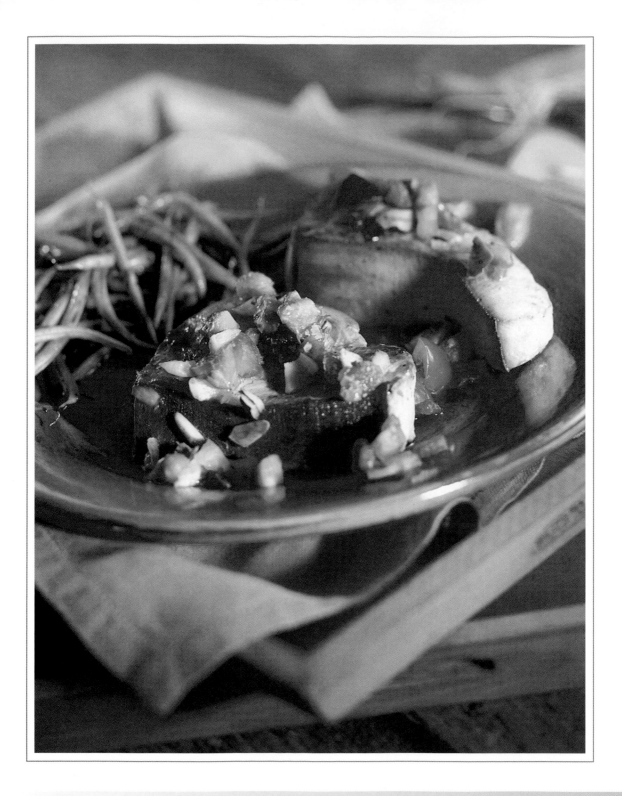

Seafood for All Occasions

Swordfish with Papaya Relish

serves 4

PER SERVING

167 calories

4.7 g. fat
(26% of calories)

0.7 g. dietary fiber

45 mg. cholesterol

339 mg. sodium

In this easy, quick-cooking dish, the delicate flavor of swordfish is enhanced by a mildly spicy sauce. Serve with steamed potatoes and cole slaw.

PREPARATION TIME
10 minutes

COOKING TIME
10 minutes

³/₄	cup diced papayas
¼	cup diced red onions
¼	cup diced green peppers
2	tablespoons chopped fresh cilantro
	Juice of 2 limes
	Salt and ground black pepper
4	swordfish steaks
4	cloves garlic, thinly sliced
1	tablespoon Asian fish sauce
1	teaspoon chopped jalapeño peppers (wear plastic gloves when handling)

In a small bowl, mix the papayas, onions, green peppers, cilantro and 2 tablespoons of the lime juice. Add salt and black pepper to taste.

In a large no-stick frying pan, combine the swordfish, garlic, fish sauce, jalapeño peppers and the remaining lime juice. Cover and cook over medium-high heat for 10 minutes, or until the fish flakes easily when tested with a fork. Serve with the papaya relish.

PREPARATION TIME
5 minutes

BAKING TIME
10 minutes

Lemon Sole with Asparagus

serves 4

This dish is light and quick—ready in 10 minutes. The asparagus cooks along with the sole and a touch of lemon and herbs.

4	sole fillets
12	asparagus spears
4	sprigs fresh marjoram
2	tablespoons chopped fresh parsley
2	tablespoons grated lemon rind

Cut 4 squares of parchment paper or aluminum foil. Place a fillet in the middle of each piece. Top with the asparagus, marjoram, parsley and lemon rind. Seal the packets. Place on a baking sheet.

Bake at 350° for 10 minutes, or until the sole flakes when tested with a fork.

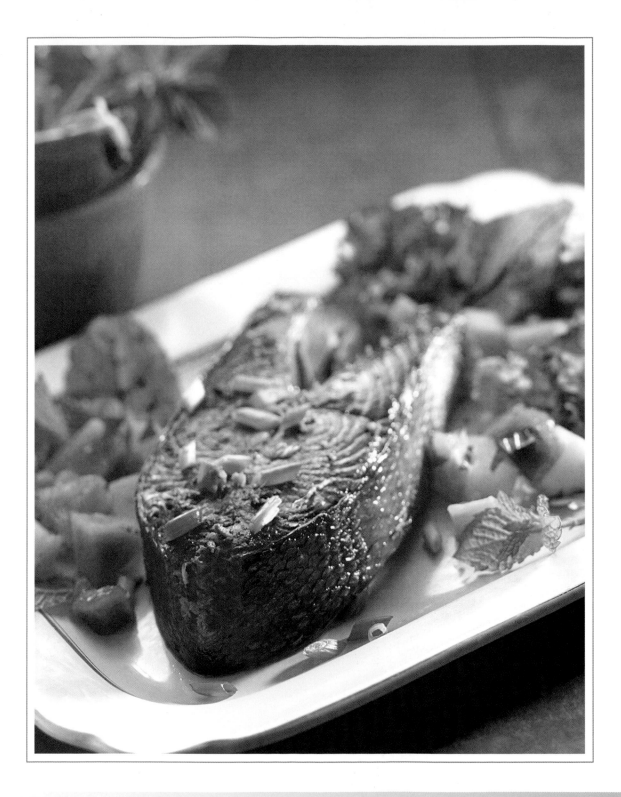

Teriyaki Salmon

serves 4

PER SERVING

183 calories

3.8 g. fat
(19% of calories)

0.1 g. dietary fiber

58 mg. cholesterol

779 mg. sodium

The flavors of the Orient inspired this simple dish. Serve with rice and cucumber salad.

$1/3$	cup reduced-sodium soy sauce
2	tablespoons mirin (rice wine) or apple juice
2	tablespoons chopped scallions
2	teaspoons grated fresh ginger
2	tablespoons honey
3	tablespoons lemon juice
4	salmon steaks

In a resealable plastic bag, mix the soy sauce, mirin or apple juice, scallions, ginger, honey and lemon juice. Add the salmon and shake well. Refrigerate for 30 minutes, turning occasionally.

Coat a broiler pan with no-stick spray and place the salmon on it. Transfer the marinade to a 1-quart saucepan and bring to a boil over medium-high heat. Cook, stirring occasionally, for 8 minutes, or until reduced by half.

Broil the salmon about 4" from the heat for 10 to 12 minutes, or until the fish flakes easily when tested with a fork; turn halfway through the cooking time. Serve with the reduced marinade.

PREPARATION TIME
5 minutes
plus 30 minutes
marinating time

COOKING TIME
20 minutes

PREPARATION TIME
5 minutes
plus 10 minutes
marinating time

COOKING TIME
15 minutes

Marinated Tuna on Broccoli Rabe

serves 4

Broccoli rabe is also known as broccoli raab and rapini. It's a broccoli relative whose assertive, slightly bitter flavor complements the rich-tasting tuna.

Marinated Tuna

2   tablespoons white wine vinegar

2   tablespoons chopped fresh oregano

1   tablespoon lemon juice

1   teaspoon olive oil

2   cloves garlic, minced

   Dash of hot-pepper sauce

4   tuna steaks

Broccoli Rabe

1/2   cup thinly sliced red onions

1/2   teaspoon olive oil

1   pound broccoli rabe, sliced (see note)

1/2   teaspoon sugar

TO MAKE THE MARINATED TUNA

In a medium bowl, mix the vinegar, oregano, lemon juice, oil, garlic and hot-pepper sauce. Add the tuna, turn to coat and let marinate for 10 minutes at room temperature.

Remove the tuna from the marinade; reserve the marinade. Grill or broil the tuna for 3 to 5 minutes per side, basting twice with the reserved marinade, until the tuna is no longer pink when tested with a knife. Transfer to a plate and keep warm. Save the remaining marinade.

TO MAKE THE BROCCOLI RABE

In a large no-stick frying pan over medium heat, sauté the onions in the oil for 1 to 2 minutes, or until soft. Add the broccoli rabe, sugar and any remaining marinade. Bring the marinade to a boil. Cook, stirring occasionally, for 2 minutes, or until the broccoli rabe is bright green. Serve with the tuna.

Chef's Note

Broccoli rabe has more stem and fewer florets than conventional broccoli. The stem is also less woody, so you can use more of it. To prepare, trim about 1" off the stem end, then chop or slice the remaining stalks. If broccoli rabe is not available, substitute sliced spinach, collard greens or kale.

Ginger Bass in Foil

serves 8

PER SERVING

211 calories

8.5 g. fat
(34% of calories)

1.3 g. dietary fiber

116 mg. cholesterol

123 mg. sodium

Here's a no-fuss entrée for a quick summer dinner. Try it with corn on the cob and steamed new potatoes.

PREPARATION TIME
10 minutes

COOKING TIME
20 minutes

2	thin zucchini, julienned
2	thin yellow squash, julienned
1	large carrot, julienned
2	tablespoons minced fresh ginger
8	bass fillets
1	lemon, quartered lengthwise
2	cloves garlic, minced
1/2	teaspoon ground black pepper

Cut 8 large squares of aluminum foil.

In a large bowl, mix the zucchini, yellow squash, carrots and ginger. Divide among the pieces of foil. Top with the fillets. Squeeze the lemon quarters over the fillets and sprinkle with the garlic and pepper.

Seal the packets and grill for 15 to 20 minutes, or until the bass flakes easily when tested with a fork.

Chef's Note

You may also bake the fish. Place the packets on baking sheets.
Bake at 425° for 15 to 20 minutes.

Seafood for All Occasions

Salmon with Lemon and Herbs

serves 4

PER SERVING

92 calories

4 g. fat
(40% of calories)

0.2 g. dietary fiber

15 mg. cholesterol

521 mg. sodium

PREPARATION TIME
5 minutes

COOKING TIME
10 minutes

Salmon makes such an elegant dinner, your guests will never guess how easy it was to prepare.

1	salmon fillet (12 ounces)
2	tablespoons lemon juice
1	teaspoon olive oil
3	sprigs fresh marjoram
3	sprigs fresh parsley
1	teaspoon grated lemon rind

Remove as many bones as possible from the salmon (see note). Place the salmon on a large piece of aluminum foil. In a cup, whisk together the lemon juice and oil; drizzle over the salmon. Place the marjoram and parsley on the salmon and sprinkle with the lemon rind.

Grill, covered, for 10 minutes, or until the fish is opaque and just begins to flake when tested with a fork. Remove and discard the marjoram and parsley.

Chef's Note

To remove fish bones, use a clean needle-nose pliers, blunt tweezers, a strawberry huller or a bone puller.

PREPARATION TIME
20 minutes

BAKING TIME
15 minutes

Cornmeal-Breaded Catfish with Sweet Pepper Relish

serves 4

Available throughout the year, catfish is a mild, delicate fish that blends well with the stronger flavors of Southwestern dishes. Serve this entrée with fresh green beans and sliced tomatoes.

Sweet Pepper Relish

³/₄	cup cider vinegar
2	tablespoons apple juice
2	tablespoons honey
¹/₂	cup diced sweet red peppers
¹/₂	cup diced green peppers
¹/₂	cup diced yellow peppers
¹/₃	cup thinly sliced onions
1	tablespoon chopped fresh mint

Catfish

³/₄	cup low-fat buttermilk
³/₄	cup cornmeal
1	tablespoon Cajun seafood seasoning
4	catfish fillets

TO MAKE THE SWEET PEPPER RELISH

In a 1-quart saucepan, mix the vinegar, apple juice and honey. Stir in the red peppers, green peppers, yellow peppers and onions. Bring to a boil over medium-high heat and cook for 1 minute, or until the onions are wilted. Stir in the mint. Remove from the heat.

TO MAKE THE CATFISH

Place the buttermilk in a shallow dish. Mix the cornmeal and Cajun seasoning on a piece of wax paper. Dip the fillets in the buttermilk and then in the cornmeal, coating each fillet thoroughly.

Line a baking sheet with aluminum foil and coat with no-stick spray. Place the fillets on the sheet and coat lightly with no-stick spray. Bake at 475° for 10 to 15 minutes, or until lightly browned and the fish flakes when tested with a fork.

Strain excess liquid from the relish and serve with the fillets.

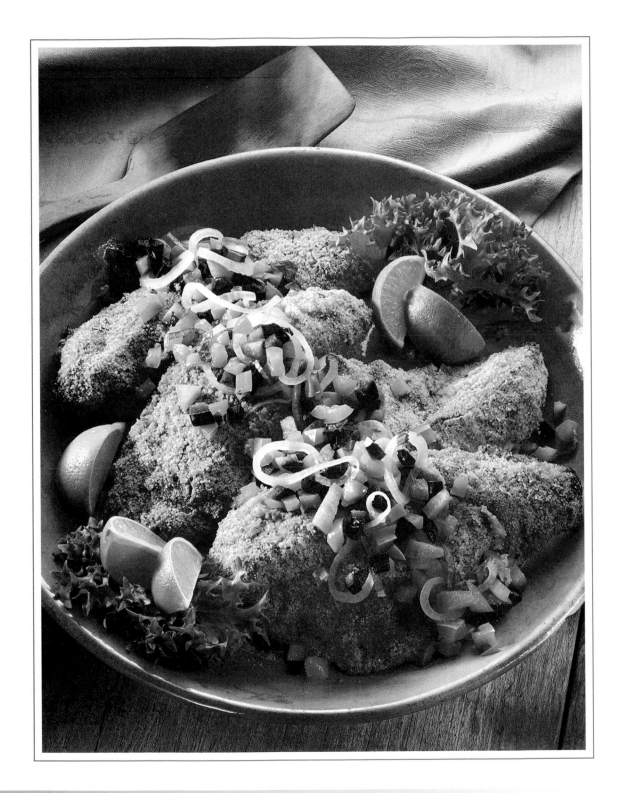

PER SERVING

254 calories

5.4 g. fat
(19% of calories)

4.9 g. dietary fiber

65 mg. cholesterol

35 mg. sodium

PREPARATION TIME
5 minutes

BAKING TIME
12 minutes

Trout with Barley, Peppers and Pine Nuts

serves 4

Barley often takes a back seat to rice and pasta in many households, but it's a deliciously nutty, nutrient-dense grain that your family will love. Quick-cooking barley takes only 10 minutes to prepare.

2	cups cooked barley
1/2	cup finely diced red peppers
2	tablespoons chopped fresh parsley
1	tablespoon toasted pine nuts
1	teaspoon grated orange rind
	Dash of hot-pepper sauce
	Salt and ground black pepper
4	trout fillets
1/4	cup fresh orange juice

In a large bowl, mix the barley, red peppers, parsley, pine nuts, orange rind and hot-pepper sauce. Add salt and black pepper to taste.

Coat an 11" × 7" baking dish with no-stick spray. Spread the barley mixture evenly in the dish. Top with the trout. Drizzle with the orange juice. Cover and bake at 400° for 8 to 12 minutes, or until the fish is opaque and flakes when tested with a fork.

Stuffed Flounder Florentine

serves 4

PER SERVING

153 calories

1.5 g. fat
(9% of calories)

1.8 g. dietary fiber

56 mg. cholesterol

183 mg. sodium

Flounder is prized for its fine texture and delicate flavor. It is sometimes mislabeled as sole, but only Dover sole is the real thing—the rest is actually flounder.

PREPARATION TIME
10 minutes

BAKING TIME
15 minutes

1	box (10 ounces) frozen chopped spinach, thawed and squeezed dry
½	cup fat-free ricotta cheese
¼	cup dry bread crumbs
2	tablespoons fat-free sour cream
2	tablespoons chopped onions
¼	teaspoon ground nutmeg
	Dash of hot-pepper sauce
	Salt and ground black pepper
4	flounder fillets
2	tablespoons orange juice

In a medium bowl, mix the spinach, ricotta, bread crumbs, sour cream, onions, nutmeg and hot-pepper sauce. Add salt and pepper to taste.

Spread the spinach mixture over the fillets to about ½" from the edge. Starting at the thin end, roll up the fillets. Secure with toothpicks.

Coat an 11" × 7" baking dish with no-stick spray. Place the fillets in the dish and drizzle with the orange juice.

Bake at 350° for 15 minutes, or until the fish is opaque and flakes when tested with a fork.

PREPARATION TIME
10 minutes
plus 20 minutes
marinating time

COOKING TIME
10 minutes

Grilled Swordfish Kabobs

serves 4

The meaty texture of swordfish makes it ideal for grilling. Other fish that would work well in this recipe are tuna, halibut and mako shark.

1/4	cup defatted chicken broth
1	tablespoon drained green peppercorns, crushed
1	teaspoon olive oil
1	teaspoon lemon juice
1 1/4	pounds swordfish steak
1	green pepper
1	lemon
8	cherry tomatoes

In a medium bowl, mix the broth, peppercorns, oil and lemon juice. Cut the swordfish into 20 equal cubes. Add to the bowl and stir to coat. Cover and refrigerate for 20 minutes to marinate.

Cut the green pepper into 1 1/2" pieces. Cut the lemon in half lengthwise, then crosswise into 1/2" slices.

Remove the fish from the marinade; reserve the marinade. Thread the peppers, swordfish, lemon slices and tomatoes onto 4 metal skewers, dividing the ingredients evenly among the skewers. Brush with the reserved marinade and grill for 6 to 10 minutes, turning once. Discard the remaining marinade.

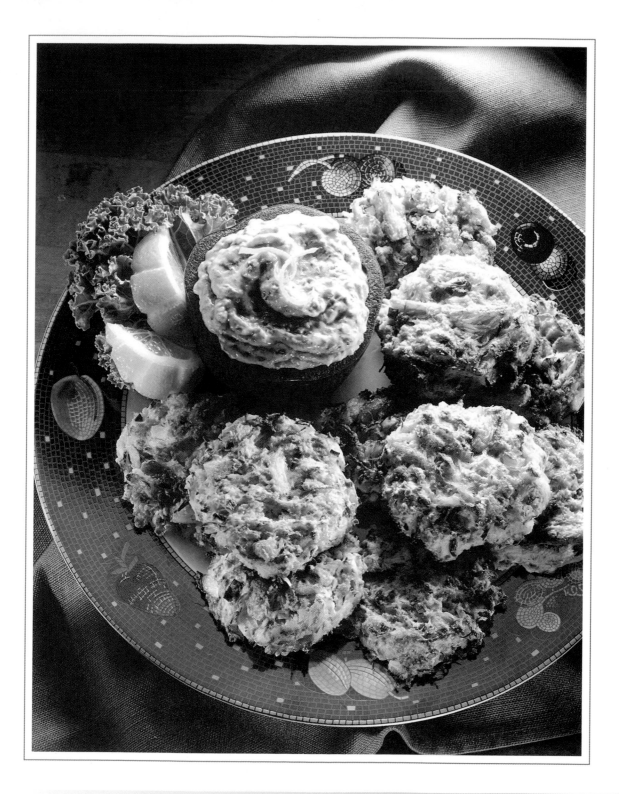

Seafood for All Occasions

Chesapeake Bay Crab Cakes with Red Pepper Tartar Sauce

serves 4

PER SERVING

247 calories

8.8 g. fat
(33% of calories)

0.4 g. dietary fiber

108 mg. cholesterol

537 mg. sodium

Maryland and the Chesapeake Bay region are renowned for their crab cakes, which are crispy on the outside and tender on the inside.

PREPARATION TIME
10 minutes

COOKING TIME
8 minutes

Crab Cakes

2	egg whites
1	tablespoon lemon juice
1/4	teaspoon dry mustard
1/4	teaspoon hot-pepper sauce
1/4	teaspoon Worcestershire sauce
1	pound crabmeat, well-drained
1/4	cup minced onions
3	tablespoons thinly sliced scallions
1/2	cup crushed oyster crackers
1/4	cup reduced-fat mayonnaise

Red Pepper Tartar Sauce

1/2	cup fat-free plain yogurt
1/4	cup minced sweet red peppers
2	tablespoons minced onions
1/8	teaspoon ground red pepper

TO MAKE THE CRAB CAKES
In a medium bowl, mix the egg whites, lemon juice, mustard, hot-pepper sauce and Worcestershire sauce. Add the crabmeat, onions and scallions and stir gently. Stir in the oyster crackers and mayonnaise. Form into 12 patties.

Line a baking sheet with aluminum foil and coat with no-stick spray. Place the patties on the sheet. Broil about 3" from the heat for 5 to 8 minutes, or until lightly browned, turning once.

TO MAKE THE RED PEPPER TARTAR SAUCE
In a food processor, process the yogurt, red peppers, onions and ground red pepper until smooth. Serve with the crab cakes.

Chef's Note

Drain the crabmeat thoroughly, pressing it in a sieve to remove extra liquid.

PREPARATION TIME
10 minutes
plus 5 minutes
marinating time

BAKING TIME
10 minutes

Baked Red Snapper

serves 4

Flavors synonymous with southern Italy—capers, olives, garlic and basil—make this fish especially good. This is delicious served with simple roasted potatoes.

1	pound red snapper fillets
1/2	cup white wine or vegetable broth
1/4	cup lemon juice
1/2	cup canned tomatoes, drained and chopped
1/4	cup chopped fresh parsley
1	teaspoon chopped fresh marjoram
1	clove garlic, minced
2	black olives, pitted and chopped
1	teaspoon drained capers
2	tablespoons chopped fresh basil

Place the snapper, skin side down, in a 13" × 9" baking dish. Pour the wine or broth and lemon juice over the fish and let marinate for 5 minutes.

Distribute the tomatoes, parsley, marjoram and garlic evenly over the snapper. Cover the dish loosely with aluminum foil. Bake at 450° for 10 minutes, or until the fish is opaque and flakes when tested with a fork. Sprinkle with the olives, capers and basil.

Chef's Note
You may also use halibut, cod or swordfish fillets in this dish.

Provençal Tuna Loaf

serves 4

PER SERVING

356 calories

7.7 g. fat
(19% of calories)

1.8 g. dietary fiber

17 mg. cholesterol

552 mg. sodium

This is perfect picnic fare. A loaf of crusty bread is hollowed out and stuffed with a savory mixture of tuna and vegetables. You can prepare it ahead and keep it chilled until needed.

PREPARATION TIME
10 minutes
plus 15 minutes
standing time

1	small round loaf crusty Italian bread
1	tablespoon olive oil
2	tablespoons balsamic vinegar
1	garlic clove, halved
1/8	teaspoon crushed red-pepper flakes
1	teaspoon dried thyme
1	jar (7 ounces) roasted sweet red peppers, drained
1	can (7 ounces) tuna packed in water, drained
1	large tomato, thinly sliced
1/2	cup thinly sliced red onions
1	teaspoon drained capers
1	cup watercress or small lettuce leaves
	Salt and ground black pepper

Halve the bread horizontally; remove the soft crumbs from inside the top half and reserve for another use. Brush the cut sides of both halves with the oil and vinegar, then rub with the cut garlic. Sprinkle with the red-pepper flakes and thyme.

On the bottom half of the loaf, layer the red peppers, tuna, tomatoes, onions, capers and watercress or lettuce. Sprinkle with the salt and black pepper. Press the top half of the loaf over the filling; wrap tightly in plastic wrap. Let it stand at room temperature for 15 minutes for the flavors to blend; slice into wedges.

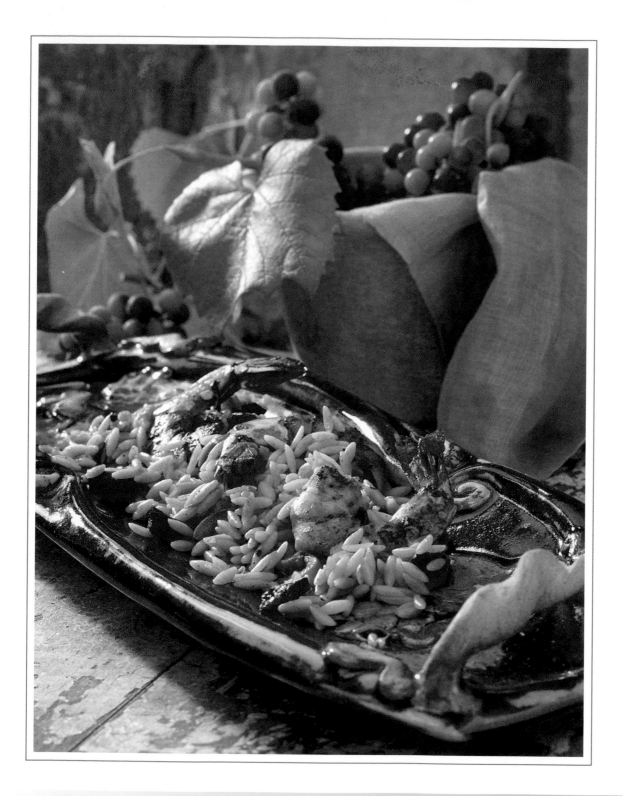

Seafood for All Occasions

Grilled Shrimp with Orzo

serves 4

Orzo pasta cooks very quickly, making it a good choice for weeknight meals. Here, it pairs with spicy marinated shrimp.

PER SERVING

351 calories

3.3 g. fat
(9% of calories)

1.2 g. dietary fiber

131 mg. cholesterol

456 mg. sodium

2	tablespoons reduced-sodium soy sauce
1	tablespoon rice vinegar
2	tablespoons honey
1	teaspoon cornstarch
2	teaspoons sesame oil
12	ounces medium shrimp, peeled and deveined
1	cup orzo
1/4	cup defatted chicken broth
1	tablespoon minced garlic
2	teaspoons chopped fresh ginger
1/4	cup sliced scallions
1/2–1	teaspoon minced jalapeño peppers (wear plastic gloves when handling)
1/2	cup shredded carrots
1/2	cup diced sweet red peppers

PREPARATION TIME
10 minutes
plus 15 minutes
marinating time

COOKING TIME
15 minutes

In a resealable plastic bag, mix the soy sauce, vinegar, honey, cornstarch, oil and shrimp. Shake well. Refrigerate for 15 minutes, turning occasionally.

Remove the shrimp, reserving the marinade. Grill the shrimp for 3 minutes, or until pink.

Cook the orzo in a pot of boiling water according to the package directions. Drain.

Bring the broth to a boil in a large no-stick frying pan over medium-high heat. Add the garlic, ginger, scallions, jalapeño peppers, carrots and red peppers. Cook for 2 to 3 minutes. Add the orzo, grilled shrimp and reserved marinade. Bring to a boil. Cook for 1 to 2 minutes, or until the sauce thickens.

PREPARATION TIME
15 minutes

COOKING TIME
10 minutes

Grilled Shrimp
with Potatoes, Peas and Basil

serves 4

Just right for languid summer appetites, this dish may be made ahead or tossed together minutes before serving.

1	pound jumbo shrimp, unpeeled
1/2	cup orange juice
1	tablespoon lemon juice
1	tablespoon white wine vinegar
1	teaspoon olive oil
1/2	teaspoon drained green peppercorns
1/4	teaspoon sugar
	Dash of hot-pepper sauce
8	new red potatoes, steamed and quartered
1	cup cooked peas
1/4	cup chopped scallions
2	tablespoons minced fresh basil
	Salt and ground black pepper

Lightly coat the shrimp with no-stick spray. Grill for 3 to 5 minutes per side, or until the shrimp turn pink. Remove the shells and devein. Set aside.

In a large bowl, whisk together the orange juice, lemon juice, vinegar, oil, peppercorns, sugar and hot-pepper sauce.

Add the potatoes, peas, scallions, basil and shrimp. Toss gently to combine. Add salt and black pepper to taste.

Chef's Note

Green peppercorns are deliciously peppery and salty-sour.
They come packed in a brine. You may omit them or replace them with capers.

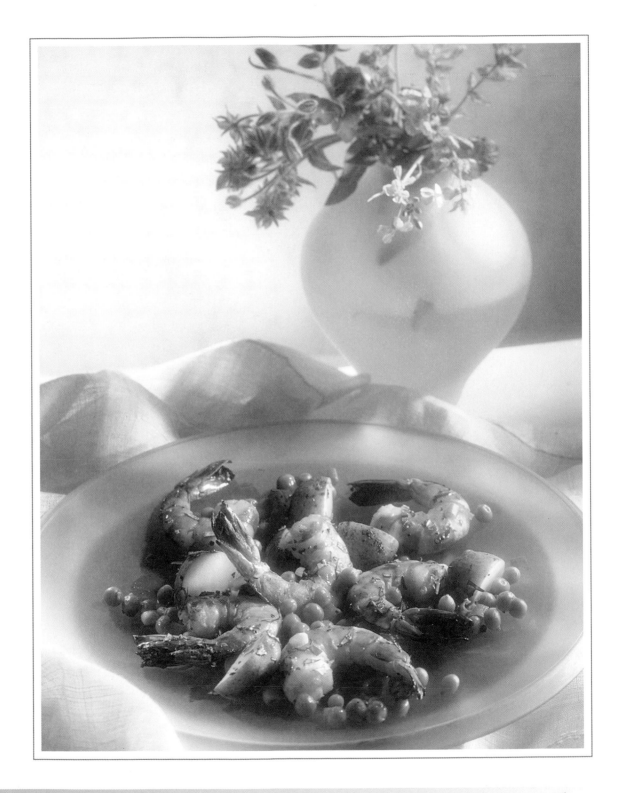

PREPARATION TIME
15 minutes

Crab Orzo Salad with Basil and Mint

serves 4

Light and refreshing, this crab and pasta salad may be made several hours ahead and kept in the refrigerator until dinnertime. Orzo is rice-shaped pasta; you may substitute other small pasta.

1/3	cup fat-free plain yogurt
1/4	cup fat-free mayonnaise
2	tablespoons lemon juice
2	tablespoons chopped fresh basil
2	tablespoons chopped fresh mint
2	cups cooked orzo
12	ounces crabmeat, well-drained
1/2	cup finely chopped sweet red peppers
1/4	cup chopped scallions
2	tablespoons toasted pine nuts

In a large bowl, whisk together the yogurt, mayonnaise, lemon juice, basil and mint. Add the orzo, crabmeat, red peppers and scallions. Mix gently. Sprinkle with the pine nuts.

Chef's Note

This dish is especially bright and attractive served in hollowed-out sweet red, yellow and orange peppers.

Spicy Jumbo Shrimp

serves 4

PER SERVING

123 calories

2.1 g. fat
(16% of calories)

0.1 g. dietary fiber

174 mg. cholesterol

201 mg. sodium

It's the chili peppers and hot-pepper sauce that give this shrimp its piquant flavor. Serve hot with rice or oven fries. Or serve cold on a bed of lettuce.

1	pound jumbo shrimp, peeled and deveined
1	teaspoon olive oil
1/2	cup white wine or water
2	tablespoons lemon juice
1	small jalapeño pepper, finely chopped (wear plastic gloves when handling)
	Dash of hot-pepper sauce

PREPARATION TIME
10 minutes

COOKING TIME
7 minutes

In a large no-stick frying pan over medium-high heat, sauté the shrimp in the oil for 1 minute. Add the wine or water, lemon juice, peppers and hot-pepper sauce. Cover and cook for 3 minutes, or until the shrimp turn pink.

Using a slotted spoon, transfer the shrimp to a serving bowl. Cook the sauce over high heat for 3 minutes, or until it is slightly reduced. Pour over the shrimp. Serve warm or cold.

PREPARATION TIME
5 minutes

COOKING TIME
10 minutes

Mussels Marinara

serves 4

Mussels are a wonderful source of iron and protein. Serve this as a main dish on a bed of pasta or as a hearty first course with crusty bread.

1/4	cup chopped onions
2	cloves garlic, minced
1	teaspoon olive oil
1	can (14 1/2 ounces) no-salt-added tomatoes, chopped (with juice)
1/3	cup white wine or clam juice
1	tablespoon lemon juice
1	tablespoon chopped fresh parsley
2	teaspoons chopped fresh oregano
1	pound mussels, scrubbed and debearded (see note)

In a large no-stick frying pan over medium heat, sauté the onions and garlic in the oil for 1 minute, or until tender. Add the tomatoes (with juice), wine or clam juice, lemon juice, parsley and oregano. Add the mussels. Cover and cook for 10 minutes, or until the mussels have opened. Discard any mussels that have not opened.

Chef's Note

To prepare mussels for cooking, scrub them under cold running water. Discard any that are already open or have broken shells. Remove the "beard" (the clump of strong, dark material that clings to the shell) from each mussel by tugging it off with your fingers or clipping it off. Don't debeard mussels until right before cooking or they will die and spoil.

Steamed Mussels with Tomatoes and Saffron

serves 4

Saffron complements the subtle flavor of mussels. Although saffron is expensive, you need only a small amount for big impact.

PER SERVING

214 calories

6.5 g. fat
(27% of calories)

2.4 g. dietary fiber

63 mg. cholesterol

588 mg. sodium

PREPARATION TIME
10 minutes

COOKING TIME
25 minutes

1 1/2	cups diced onions
1	tablespoon olive oil
4	cloves garlic, minced
2	cans (14 1/2 ounces each) no-salt-added tomatoes, drained and chopped
2	cups defatted chicken broth
1/2	teaspoon saffron threads, crushed
4	dozen large mussels, scrubbed and debearded (see note on page 184)

In a soup pot over medium heat, sauté the onions in the oil for 5 minutes, or until the onions begin to wilt. Add the garlic and sauté for 30 seconds. Add the tomatoes, broth and saffron. Bring to a boil. Partially cover the pot, reduce the heat and simmer for 10 minutes.

Add the mussels. Cover and cook over high heat for 10 minutes, or until the mussels open; shake the pot occasionally. Discard any mussels that have not opened. Serve the mussels in shallow bowls and spoon the tomato mixture over them.

PREPARATION TIME
15 minutes

COOKING TIME
30 minutes

Seafood Creole

serves 4

New Orleans and the bayou country of Louisiana are the birthplace of Creole cooking. In this recipe, fresh shrimp and fish pair with a spicy sauce.

2	cups diced onions
1	teaspoon olive oil
1	green pepper, diced
3/4	cup diced celery
3	cloves garlic, minced
2	cans (14 1/2 ounces each) no-salt-added tomatoes, chopped
1	teaspoon dried thyme
1	bay leaf
1/4	teaspoon ground red pepper
8	ounces medium shrimp, peeled and deveined
8	ounces cod or orange roughy fillets, cut into 1" pieces
2	cups hot cooked rice

In a soup pot over medium-high heat, sauté the onions in the oil for 2 minutes. Add the green peppers and celery; cook for 2 minutes. Add the garlic; cook for 1 minute.

Add the tomatoes (with juice), thyme, bay leaf and red pepper. Bring to a boil. Reduce the heat to medium and simmer for 15 to 20 minutes, or until the vegetables are just tender.

Add the shrimp and fish. Cover and cook for 3 to 5 minutes, or until the shrimp turns pink and the fish is opaque.

Remove and discard the bay leaf. Serve the shrimp mixture over the rice.

Cape Cod Scallops with Tomatoes

serves 4

PREPARATION TIME
10 minutes

COOKING TIME
20 minutes

This dish has the consistency of a chunky stew. Serve it over rice or pasta.

2	cups sliced mushrooms
1	cup sliced onions
1	teaspoon olive oil
1½	cups diced tomatoes
1	cup defatted chicken broth
1¼	pounds sea scallops
3	tablespoons minced fresh parsley
2	tablespoons lemon juice
½	teaspoon dried basil
¼	teaspoon dried rosemary
1	clove garlic, minced

In a large no-stick frying pan over medium-high heat, sauté the mushrooms and onions in the oil for 5 minutes. Add the tomatoes and broth. Bring to a boil.

Add the scallops, parsley, lemon juice, basil, rosemary and garlic. Reduce the heat and simmer for 5 minutes, or until the scallops are opaque. Using a slotted spoon, transfer the scallops and vegetables to a serving bowl.

Raise the heat to high and boil the stock for 5 minutes, or until reduced by half. Pour over the scallop mixture.

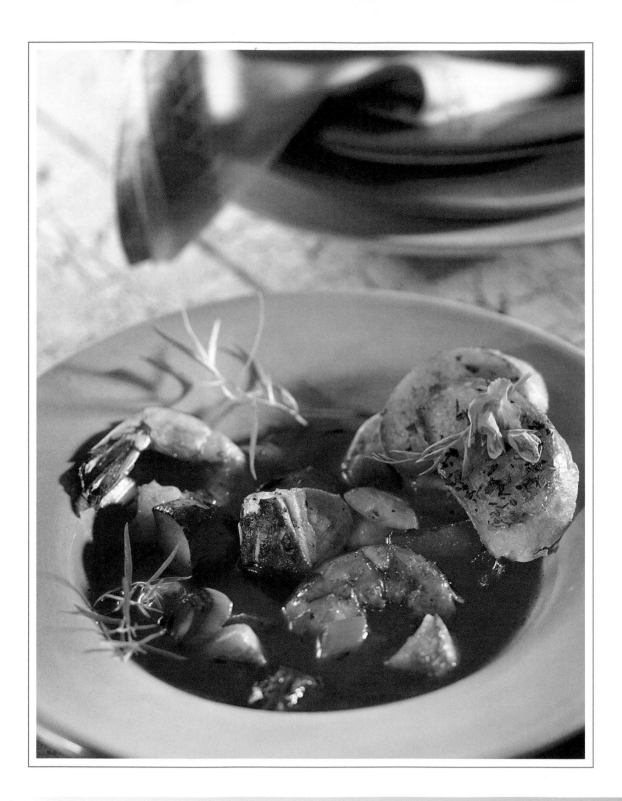

Bouillabaisse

serves 4

Bouillabaisse is a traditional French stew brimming with seafood. It's ideal for wintry evenings, served in crockery bowls with crunchy toast and a tossed salad.

1	tablespoon olive oil
2	bottles (8 ounces each) clam juice
1	cup chopped onions
2	leeks, thinly sliced
5	cloves garlic, minced
12	ounces small red potatoes, quartered
1	can (28 ounces) chopped Italian plum tomatoes (with juice)
1	pound halibut, cut into 2" cubes
8	ounces bay scallops
8	ounces large shrimp, peeled and deveined
2–3	tablespoons chopped fresh tarragon or basil
	Salt and ground black pepper

In a soup pot over medium-high heat, bring the oil and ¼ cup of the clam juice to a boil. Add the onions, leeks, garlic and potatoes. Cook for 3 to 5 minutes, or until the onions are lightly browned. Add the tomatoes (with juice); bring to a boil. Cook for 10 minutes.

Add the halibut, scallops and shrimp. Cook for 5 minutes, or until the fish is opaque and flakes easily when tested with a fork. Stir in the tarragon or basil. Add salt and pepper to taste.

PER SERVING

420 calories

7.9 g. fat
(17% of calories)

3.4 g. dietary fiber

148 mg. cholesterol

474 mg. sodium

PREPARATION TIME
10 minutes

COOKING TIME
20 minutes

chapter 7

Meaty Entrées

BEEF, PORK AND LAMB RECIPES THAT CAN'T MISS

The heartland of America raises some of the best beef, pork and lamb in the world. But it's far different from the meat that our grandparents remember. Producers heard the consumer speak, and the consumer said, "I want less fat in my meat." So today's cuts are lean and meaty but just as versatile as ever. There are even new cuts that are especially lean but also tender. So don't feel guilty about enjoying meat. Eat it often in low-fat versions of favorites like steak sandwiches, beef stew, pork and sauerkraut, pork barbecue and curried lamb.

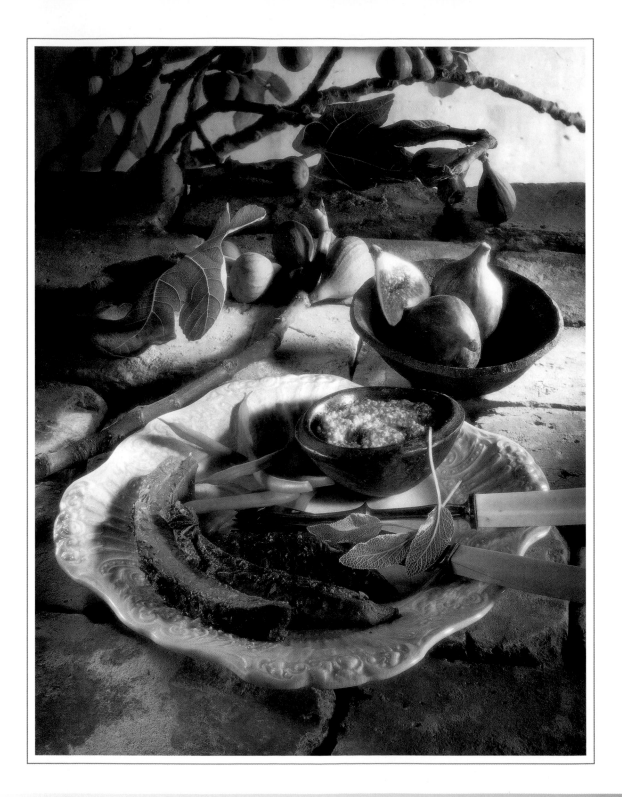

Marinated Tuscan Steak

serves 4

A simple marinade complements the rich flavors of flank steak, a lean and inexpensive cut of meat. It is just right served alongside baked potatoes. Leftovers are delicious in a salad or sandwich with sharp mustard.

2	cups orange juice
2	tablespoons grated orange rind
2	tablespoons chopped fresh sage
2	tablespoons red wine vinegar
3	cloves garlic, minced
1	teaspoon Dijon mustard
1	teaspoon ground black pepper
1	pound flank steak

In a large bowl, mix the orange juice, orange rind, sage, vinegar, garlic, mustard and pepper. Add the steak and turn to coat. Refrigerate for 15 minutes or up to 24 hours, turning occasionally.

Remove the steak from the marinade and broil about 5" from the heat for 5 minutes per side, or until the meat is light pink when tested with a knife for medium-rare. Baste twice with the marinade while broiling; discard the remaining marinade.

To serve, slice thinly across the grain and on an angle.

Chef's Note
This marinade is also good with chicken breasts and turkey tenderloins.

PER SERVING

183 calories

8 g. fat
(40% of calories)

0 g. dietary fiber

52 mg. cholesterol

71 mg. sodium

PREPARATION TIME
5 minutes
plus 15 minutes
marinating time

COOKING TIME
10 minutes

PREPARATION TIME
10 minutes

COOKING TIME
1¾ hours

Old-Fashioned Pot Roast

serves 6

Here's a slimmed-down version of an all-American favorite. Leftovers are great for sandwiches and super-quick dinners.

1	beef top round roast (1½ pounds), trimmed of all visible fat
1	cup tomato juice
½	cup red wine or defatted beef broth
1	tablespoon Dijon mustard
1	teaspoon dried rosemary
1	pound baby carrots
12	ounces new red potatoes, peeled
8	small onions
3	stalks celery, sliced into 1" pieces

Lightly coat a Dutch oven with no-stick spray. Add the beef and brown on all sides over medium-high heat. Transfer the beef to a plate. Add the tomato juice, wine or broth, mustard and rosemary to the pot. Mix well and bring to a boil over high heat. Return the beef to the pot.

Cover and bake at 325° for 45 minutes. Add the carrots, potatoes, onions and celery. Cover and bake for 45 to 60 minutes, or until the beef is tender.

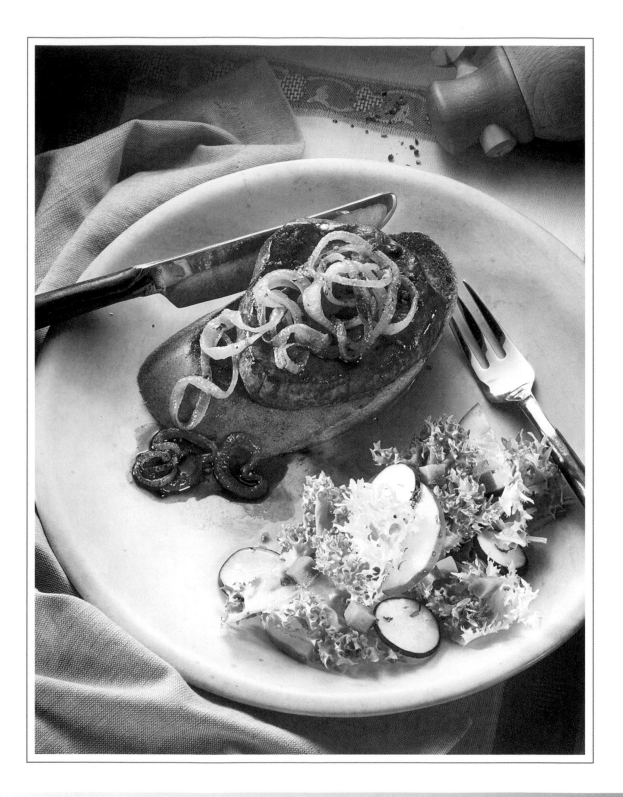

Meaty Entrées

Beef and Caramelized Onions

serves 4

PER SERVING

286 calories

9.4 g. fat
(30% of calories)

1.9 g. dietary fiber

58 mg. cholesterol

299 mg. sodium

Caramelizing onions brings out a sweet, mild flavor that complements these lean steaks.

Caramelized Onions

2	cups sliced onions
2	teaspoons canola oil
1/2	cup defatted beef broth
1/2	tablespoon brown sugar
1	tablespoon balsamic vinegar

Steaks

4	tenderloin or top round steaks (3 ounces each), trimmed of all visible fat
1/4	teaspoon cracked black pepper
4	shallots, sliced
4	cloves garlic, sliced
1/2	cup defatted beef broth
1	teaspoon red wine vinegar
4	slices sourdough bread, grilled or broiled

PREPARATION TIME
15 minutes

COOKING TIME
30 minutes

TO MAKE THE CARAMELIZED ONIONS
In a large no-stick frying pan over medium-high heat, cook the onions in the oil for 5 to 7 minutes, or until brown. Add the broth, brown sugar and vinegar. Cook for 10 to 15 minutes, or until all the liquid evaporates. Transfer to a plate.

TO MAKE THE STEAKS
In the same frying pan over medium-high heat, sear the steaks for 1 to 2 minutes per side. Season with the pepper. Reduce the heat to medium and add the shallots and garlic. Cook for 5 minutes. Add the broth and vinegar. Bring to a boil. Cook for 1 to 2 minutes, or until the steaks are cooked through and no longer pink when tested with a knife.

Serve over the bread and top with the onions.

PREPARATION TIME
10 minutes

COOKING TIME
15 minutes

Philadelphia Steak Sandwiches

serves 4

Rocky Balboa, the boxer-hero of the movies, introduced millions of Americans to Philadelphia's beloved steak sandwich. This low-fat version features reduced-fat mozzarella and plenty of sautéed vegetables. If you're adventuresome, add zing with hot cherry peppers.

1	sweet red pepper, diced
1	green pepper, diced
1	medium onion, diced
8	mushrooms, thinly sliced
2	tablespoons sliced garlic
12	ounces beef round tip steak, sliced paper thin (see note)
¼	cup ketchup
1	teaspoon dried oregano
¼	teaspoon ground black pepper
1	cup shredded reduced-fat mozzarella cheese
4	steak rolls, split and warmed

Coat a large no-stick frying pan with no-stick spray and warm over medium-high heat for 2 minutes. Add the sweet red peppers, green peppers, onions and mushrooms. Sauté for 5 minutes, or until browned.

Add the garlic and steak. Sauté for 3 minutes, or until the steak is no longer pink. Stir in the ketchup, oregano and black pepper. Sprinkle with the mozzarella. Cover and cook over low heat for 5 minutes, or until the mozzarella melts. Divide among the rolls.

Chef's Note
Freezing the steak for about 20 minutes will firm it enough to make thin-slicing easier.

Spicy Beef Burgers

Serves 4

Nothing could be faster or easier for summer weeknight dinners.

1	pound extra-lean ground round
2	tablespoons barbecue sauce
1	tablespoon steak sauce
1	tablespoon minced garlic
1	tablespoon chopped jalapeño peppers (wear plastic gloves when handling)
1	teaspoon chili powder
4	hamburger buns, split
1	tablespoon fat-free mayonnaise

In a medium bowl, mix the beef, barbecue sauce, steak sauce, garlic, peppers and chili powder. Form into 4 patties. Grill for 4 minutes per side, or until cooked through.

Toast the buns, spread with the mayonnaise and top with the patties.

PER SERVING

261 calories

6.7 g. fat
(23% of calories)

0.3 g. dietary fiber

55 mg. cholesterol

400 mg. sodium

PREPARATION TIME
5 minutes

COOKING TIME
8 minutes

PREPARATION TIME
15 minutes

COOKING TIME
10 minutes

Texas Beef Soft Tacos

Serves 4

By using soft flour tortillas instead of fried corn shells, we cut fat on this Tex-Mex favorite.

12	ounces beef tenderloin, trimmed of all visible fat
1½	teaspoons ground cumin
¼	cup defatted chicken broth
1	cup chopped sweet red peppers
3	cloves garlic, minced
2	canned chipotle chili peppers in adobo sauce, minced
½	cup mild salsa
8	large flour tortillas
3	ounces shredded reduced-fat Monterey Jack cheese
¼	cup fat-free sour cream
¼	cup chopped fresh cilantro

Cut the beef across the grain into very thin strips. Place in a large bowl, sprinkle with the cumin and toss well.

Bring the broth to a boil in a large no-stick frying pan over medium-high heat. Add the red peppers and garlic; cook for 3 minutes. Transfer to a plate. Add the beef to the pan and cook for 5 minutes. Stir in the chili peppers, salsa and the red pepper mixture. Cook for 2 minutes.

Wrap the tortillas in plastic wrap and microwave on high power for 1 minute. Divide the beef mixture among the tortillas, top with the Monterey Jack, sour cream and cilantro. Roll up.

Sweet Potato Salad recipe on page 114

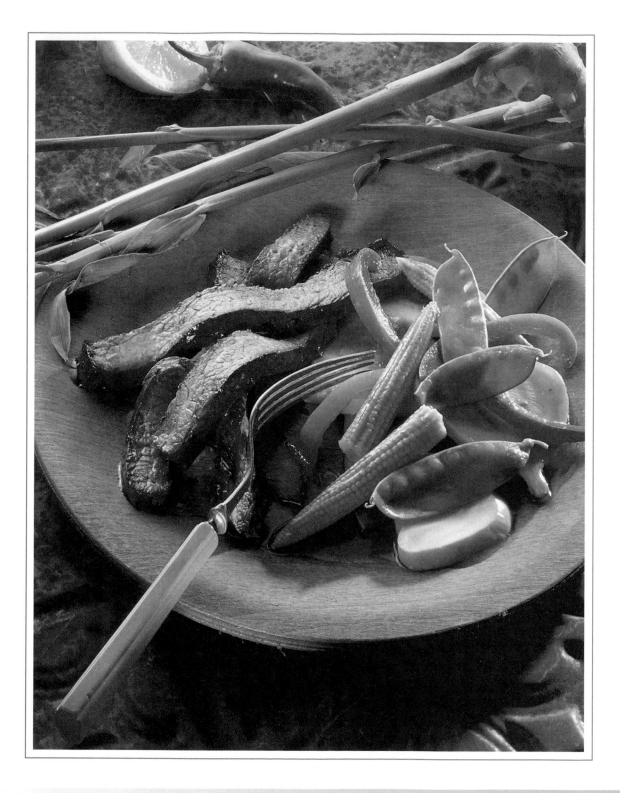

Meaty Entrées

Grilled Marinated Flank Steak

Serves 4

Flank steak is very lean, yet it's often overlooked because it can be tough. This recipe keeps it moist and tender by marinating it and then cooking it very quickly on the grill.

PER SERVING

218 calories

8.2 g. fat
(35% of calories)

0 g. dietary fiber

50 mg. cholesterol

589 mg. sodium

1	pound flank steak
1/4	cup lemon juice
1/4	cup reduced-sodium soy sauce
1	teaspoon minced garlic
1	teaspoon grated fresh ginger
1	teaspoon chopped jalapeño peppers (wear plastic gloves when handling)

PREPARATION TIME
5 minutes
plus 25 minutes
marinating time

COOKING TIME
14 minutes

In a resealable plastic bag, combine the steak, lemon juice, soy sauce, garlic, ginger and peppers. Shake well. Refrigerate for 25 minutes or up to 24 hours, turning occasionally.

Remove the steak from the marinade and grill for 7 minutes per side, or until the meat is light pink when tested with a knife for medium-rare. Baste twice with the marinade while grilling; discard the remaining marinade.

To serve, slice thinly across the grain and on an angle.

PREPARATION TIME
10 minutes

COOKING TIME
15 minutes

Savory Beef Stew

serves 4

Pressure cooking produces old-fashioned beef stew in record time. It's great served with noodles and green peas.

1/4	cup all-purpose flour
1/2	teaspoon salt
1/4	teaspoon dry mustard
1	pound lean sirloin, trimmed of all visible fat and cubed
1 1/2	teaspoons olive oil
1/2	cup defatted beef broth
1	can (14 ounces) tomatoes (with juice), chopped
1	cup diced red potatoes
1/2	cup diced onions
1	medium carrot, chopped
2	tablespoons minced garlic
2	tablespoons tomato paste
2	tablespoons balsamic vinegar
1	tablespoon brown sugar
1 1/2	teaspoons dried thyme
2	bay leaves

In a resealable plastic bag, combine the flour, salt, mustard and sirloin. Shake well. Warm the oil in a pressure cooker over medium-high heat. Transfer the sirloin to the pan and brown on all sides.

Add the broth and bring to a boil, scraping the bottom of the pan to loosen any browned bits. Add the tomatoes (with juice), potatoes, onions, carrots, garlic, tomato paste, vinegar, brown sugar, thyme and bay leaves.

Lock the pressure cooker lid in place and bring to high pressure over high heat. Cook for 12 minutes. Release the pressure. Remove and discard the bay leaves.

Chef's Note

If you don't have a pressure cooker, use a Dutch oven. Increase the amount of beef broth to 3 cups and cook for 1 1/2 to 2 hours over medium heat, stirring occasionally.

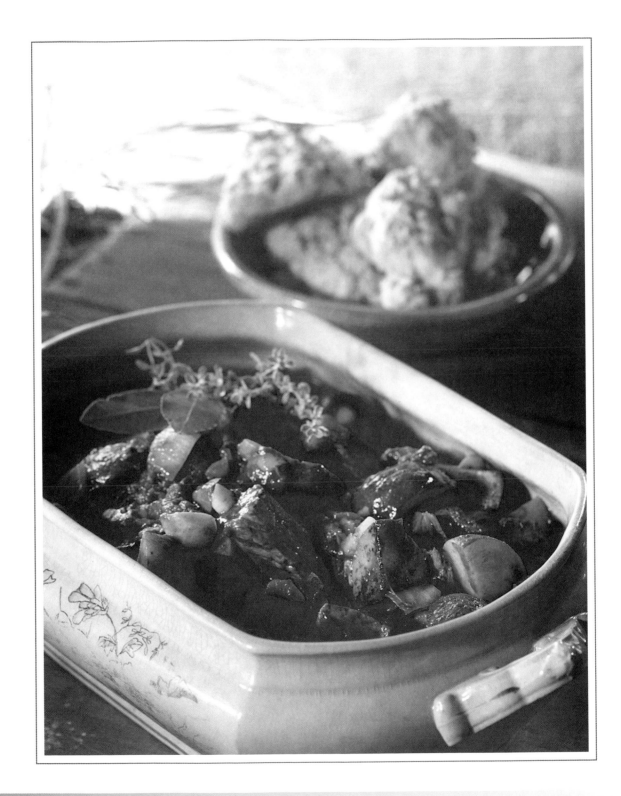

PREPARATION TIME
15 minutes
plus 25 minutes
marinating time

COOKING TIME
20 minutes

Fajitas with Coriander Cream

serves 4

Coriander is one of the herbs that gives Southwestern cooking its distinctive flavor. You can easily grow it in your backyard garden or in patio pots. In this recipe, it seasons both the marinade and the sour cream sauce.

1/2	cup lime juice
1/4	cup chopped fresh coriander
1	tablespoon minced garlic
2	teaspoons cumin seeds, crushed
1/2	teaspoon ground black pepper
12	ounces flank steak
1	cup fat-free sour cream
1/2	cup chopped fresh coriander
1/2	teaspoon grated lime rind
1	sweet red pepper, halved
1	green pepper, halved
1	onion, quartered
1	cup diced avocado
1	cup salsa
8	large flour tortillas

In a glass baking dish, mix the lime juice, coriander, garlic, cumin and pepper. Add the steak and turn to coat. Cover and refrigerate for 25 minutes or up to 24 hours, turning occasionally.

Remove the steak from the marinade and grill for 7 minutes per side, or until the meat is light pink when tested with a knife for medium-rare. Baste twice with the marinade while grilling; discard the remaining marinade.

Meanwhile, in a blender or small food processor, combine the sour cream, coriander and lime rind. Blend until smooth, stopping to scrape down the sides as needed. Set aside.

Grill the red and green peppers and the onion for 10 to 15 minutes, or until brown. Slice into thin strips.

In a small bowl, mix the avocados and salsa.

Wrap 4 of the tortillas in a paper towel and microwave on high power for 20 seconds, or until hot. Repeat with the remaining 4 tortillas.

Divide the steak among the tortillas. Top with the vegetables, coriander cream and salsa. Roll to enclose the filling.

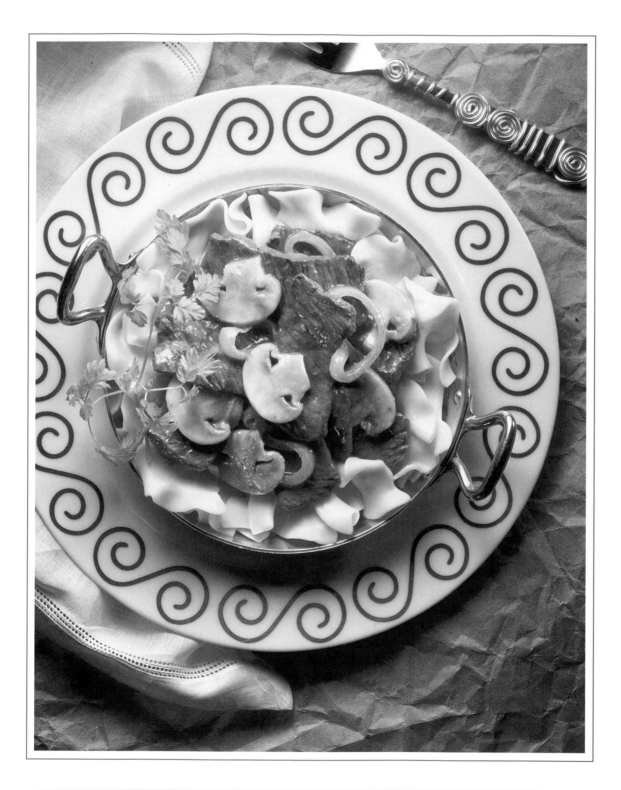

Meaty Entrées

Beef Stroganoff

serves 4

Traditional stroganoff recipes are loaded with sour cream, making them really high in calories and fat. This version is much lighter but just as satisfying.

PER SERVING

449 calories

19 g. fat
(38% of calories)

2 g. dietary fiber

101 mg. cholesterol

720 mg. sodium

PREPARATION TIME
10 minutes

COOKING TIME
15 minutes

1	pound lean sirloin, trimmed of all visible fat and cut into strips
1/2	teaspoon salt
1/4	teaspoon dry mustard
1/4	cup plus 1 tablespoon all-purpose flour
2	teaspoons olive oil
1 1/2	cups defatted beef broth
2	tablespoons balsamic vinegar
1 1/2	teaspoons dried thyme
1	large onion, sliced
8	ounces mushrooms, sliced
2	tablespoons minced garlic
2	bay leaves
8	ounces sour cream
	Salt and ground black pepper
8	ounces noodles, cooked

In a resealable plastic bag, combine the sirloin, salt, mustard and 1/4 cup of the flour. Shake well.

Warm the oil in a large no-stick frying pan over medium-high heat. Shake excess flour off the beef and add the beef to the pan. Stir to brown on all sides. Transfer to a plate.

Add the broth, vinegar and thyme to the pan. Bring to a boil, scraping the bottom of the pan to loosen any browned bits. Add the onions, mushrooms, garlic and bay leaves. Cook, stirring frequently, for 5 minutes. Add the beef. Cover, reduce the heat to low and simmer for 5 minutes.

In a small bowl, stir together the sour cream and the remaining 1 tablespoon flour. Stir into the pan and heat through. Season with the salt and pepper to taste. Remove and discard the bay leaves. Serve over the noodles.

PREPARATION TIME
5 minutes
plus 30 minutes
marinating time

COOKING TIME
10 minutes

Pork BBQ Sandwiches

Serves 4

You don't need to spend the whole day slaving over the barbecue pit to enjoy the taste of real Texas-style barbecue.

1	pound boneless pork tenderloin, cut into 4 slices
1	tablespoon chopped chipotle chili peppers in adobo sauce
1	cup plus 1 tablespoon reduced-sodium barbecue sauce
8	slices thick Italian bread, grilled

In a resealable plastic bag, combine the pork, peppers and 1 cup of the barbecue sauce. Shake well. Refrigerate for 30 minutes or up to 24 hours, turning occasionally.

Grill the pork for 5 minutes per side, or until slightly charred and no longer pink when tested with a knife. Slice thin.

Lightly grill the buns and spread the cut sides with the remaining 1 tablespoon barbecue sauce. Top with the pork.

Oven-Fried Pepper-Dusted Potato Wedges recipe on page 302

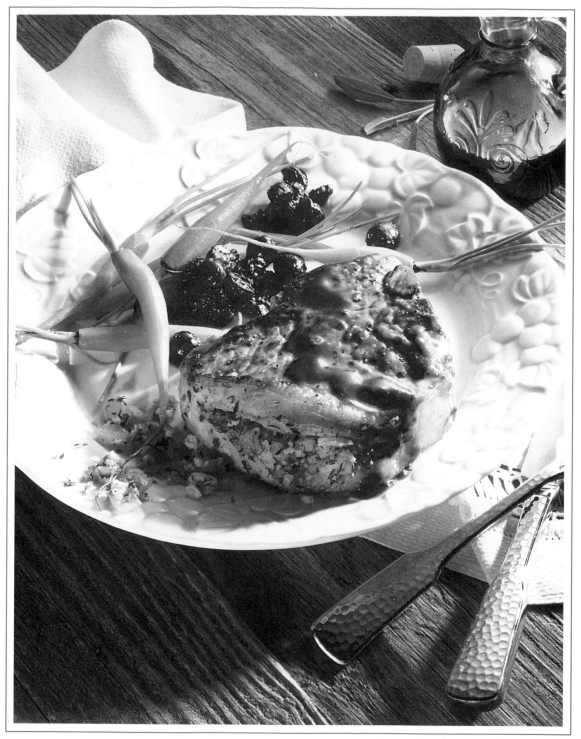

Honey-Glazed Carrots recipe on page 314

Meaty Entrées

Stuffed Pork Loin Chops

Serves 4

As good as slow-cooked pork roast but ready in a fraction of the time, these stuffed pork chops will satisfy the heartiest appetite.

PER SERVING

272 calories

11.2 g. fat
(38% of calories)

0.2 g. dietary fiber

54 mg. cholesterol

368 mg. sodium

4	thick-cut pork loin chops, trimmed of all visible fat
1½	cups dry cornbread stuffing
1	teaspoon poultry seasoning
¼	cup minced onions
2–2½	cups defatted chicken broth
2	tablespoons balsamic vinegar
1	teaspoon cornstarch
1	tablespoon water

Cut a slit in the side of each chop to form a pocket. In a small bowl, mix the stuffing, poultry seasoning, onions and ½ to 1 cup of the broth (enough to create a moist stuffing). Pack the stuffing into the pockets; seal the pockets shut with wooden toothpicks, if necessary.

Coat a large no-stick frying pan with no-stick cooking spray and place over medium-high heat for 2 minutes. Add the pork chops. Brown for 2 to 3 minutes per side. Add 1 cup of the remaining broth. Cover, reduce the heat to low and simmer for 25 minutes, or until the pork is tender and no longer pink when tested with a knife. Transfer to a plate.

Add the vinegar and the remaining ½ cup broth to the pan. Bring to a boil. In a cup, mix the cornstarch and water; add to the pan. Cook, stirring, until the broth has thickened; pour over the pork chops.

PREPARATION TIME
10 minutes

COOKING TIME
35 minutes

PREPARATION TIME
10 minutes

COOKING TIME
30 minutes

Simmered
Sauerkraut and Pork

serves 4

Bring Oktoberfest to your dining room when you serve this authentic German supper. Dark rye bread, chunky cinnamon-flavored applesauce and mashed potatoes topped with browned onions would complete the meal nicely.

½	cup dried apple slices
1	cup diced onions
3	strips turkey bacon, diced
1	teaspoon canola oil
2	cups sauerkraut, rinsed and drained
1	cup defatted chicken broth
⅛	teaspoon fennel seeds
⅛	teaspoon caraway seeds
4	pork chops (3 ounces each), trimmed of all visible fat

Place the apples in a small bowl; cover with hot water and let stand for 5 minutes. Drain.

In a Dutch oven over medium heat, sauté the onions and bacon in the oil for 5 minutes. Add the sauerkraut, broth, fennel seeds, caraway seeds and apples. Cover and simmer for 10 minutes.

Coat a large no-stick frying pan with no-stick spray and warm over medium heat. Add the pork chops and cook for 2 minutes per side, or until browned. Transfer to the Dutch oven. Cover and simmer for 10 minutes, or until the pork chops are cooked through and no longer pink when tested with a knife.

Pork Chops
with Apple Onion Relish

serves 4

PER SERVING

178 calories

7.4 g. fat
(37% of calories)

1.8 g. dietary fiber

44 mg. cholesterol

36 mg. sodium

Apples and onions are perfect partners for pork. In this recipe, they create a tangy-sweet relish that can be served hot or cold. Round out the meal with baked sweet potatoes and steamed broccoli.

4	pork chops (3 ounces each), trimmed of all visible fat
1/2	cup chopped onions
1	cinnamon stick
1/4	cup apple cider
2 1/2	cups diced Granny Smith apples
1	teaspoon cider vinegar
1	teaspoon honey

PREPARATION TIME
10 minutes

COOKING TIME
20 minutes

Coat a large no-stick frying pan with no-stick spray and warm over medium-high heat for 2 minutes. Add the pork chops and cook for 2 minutes per side, or until brown. Reduce the heat to medium and cook for 10 minutes, or until cooked through and until no longer pink when tested with a knife.

In a 2-quart saucepan, combine the onions, cinnamon stick and cider. Cook over medium-low heat for 10 minutes. Add the apples, cover and cook for 5 minutes, or until the apples are soft. Stir in the vinegar and honey. Remove and discard the cinnamon stick. Serve with the pork chops.

Chef's Note

You may use any other tart, crisp apples in this recipe. For more color, don't peel the apples and use a mixture of red and green.

PREPARATION TIME
10 minutes
plus 15 minutes
marinating time

COOKING TIME
25 minutes

Sunshine Pork

serves 4

Red grapefruit puts the sunshine in this grilled main dish. For attractive splashes of color, use a mixture of red, green and yellow sweet peppers. Serve the pork with couscous or a blend of wild and white rice.

Pork and Marinade

1	cup orange juice
2	tablespoons white wine vinegar
1	tablespoon grated orange rind
2	teaspoons minced fresh rosemary
1	pound pork tenderloin, cut into 4 pieces

Citrus Sauce

1	sweet red pepper, julienned
4	scallions, cut into 1/2" slices
2	teaspoons canola oil
1/4	cup apple cider
2	oranges, peeled and sectioned
1	red grapefruit, peeled and sectioned
1/4	teaspoon black pepper
1	teaspoon cornstarch
1	tablespoon cold water
2	teaspoons chopped fresh mint

TO MAKE THE PORK AND MARINADE
In a glass baking dish, mix the orange juice, vinegar, orange rind and rosemary. Add the pork and turn to coat. Cover and refrigerate for 15 minutes or up to 24 hours, turning occasionally.

Remove the pork from the marinade; reserve the marinade. Grill the pork for 10 to 15 minutes, or until cooked through and no longer pink when tested with a knife.

TO MAKE THE CITRUS SAUCE
In a large no-stick frying pan over medium-high heat, sauté the red peppers and scallions in the oil for 3 minutes. Add the cider, oranges, grapefruit, black pepper and reserved marinade. In a cup, mix the cornstarch and water; stir into the pan. Cook for 3 to 5 minutes, or until thickened. Pour over the pork and sprinkle with the mint.

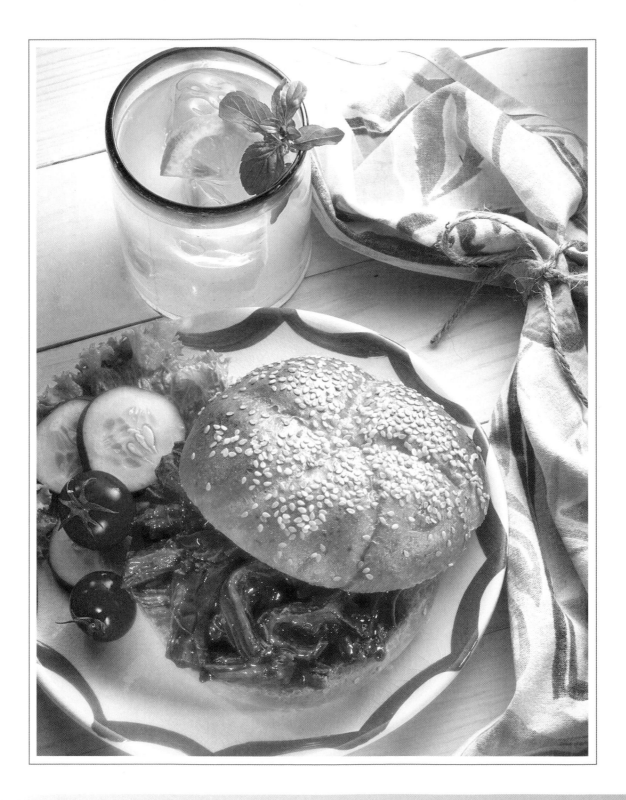

Meaty Entrées

Pulled Pork Barbecue

serves 4

You "pull" pork by shredding it with two forks. Serve this Southern-style barbecued pork on buns along with your favorite slaw, sliced tomatoes, corn on the cob and watermelon for a summer picnic.

PER SERVING

270 calories

6.4 g. fat
(22% of calories)

2.4 g. dietary fiber

60 mg. cholesterol

399 mg. sodium

PREPARATION TIME
10 minutes

COOKING TIME
45 minutes

1	chipotle pepper (wear plastic gloves when handling)
12	ounces pork tenderloin
$1/4$	teaspoon ground black pepper
$1/8$	teaspoon ground red pepper
$2/3$	cup diced onions
1	teaspoon canola oil
1	tablespoon minced garlic
$1/2$	cup barbecue sauce
$1/4$	cup ketchup
$1/4$	cup water
1	teaspoon maple syrup
4	sandwich buns, split and warmed

Place the chipotle pepper in a small bowl; cover with hot water and let stand for 5 minutes. Drain; remove the stem and seeds. Coarsely chop the pepper.

Coat a large no-stick frying pan with no-stick spray and warm over high heat. Add the pork and brown on all sides. Sprinkle with the black pepper and red pepper. Transfer to a large sheet of aluminum foil.

In a 2-quart saucepan over medium heat, sauté the onions in the oil for 5 minutes. Add the garlic and cook for 1 minute. Add the barbecue sauce, ketchup, water, maple syrup and chipotle peppers. Bring to a boil and simmer for 10 minutes.

Spoon one-third of the sauce over the pork. Wrap well and bake at 350° for 25 minutes, or until tender and no longer pink when tested with a knife.

Shred the pork using 2 forks. Add to the remaining sauce and heat through. Serve on the buns.

Chef's Note

Chipotle peppers are smoked and dried jalapeños. There is no substitute for the flavor they add, but a fresh serrano or jalapeño pepper can be used to add the same spiciness.

PREPARATION TIME
5 minutes

COOKING TIME
10 minutes

Pork with Balsamic Vinegar and Pears

serves 4

Combining pork tenderloin with pungent-sweet balsamic vinegar and sliced pears makes an elegant dinner entrée that's low in fat.

1	pound pork tenderloin, cut into 4 pieces
2	teaspoons all-purpose flour
1	cup defatted chicken broth
1/2	cup sliced scallions
1	tablespoon balsamic vinegar
1	pear, sliced

Pound the tenderloin pieces with a wooden mallet to flatten them slightly. Lightly dust with the flour and shake off any excess.

Coat a large no-stick frying pan with no-stick spray. Add the pork and brown over high heat for 2 to 3 minutes per side, or until just cooked through. Transfer to a plate.

Add the broth, scallions and vinegar to the pan. Cover, reduce the heat and simmer for 2 minutes, or until the scallions are soft. Uncover and cook for 1 to 2 minutes, or until the broth is reduced to a thin glaze.

Stir in the pears. Return the pork to the pan and heat through.

Chef's Note

An apple will also work well in this dish.

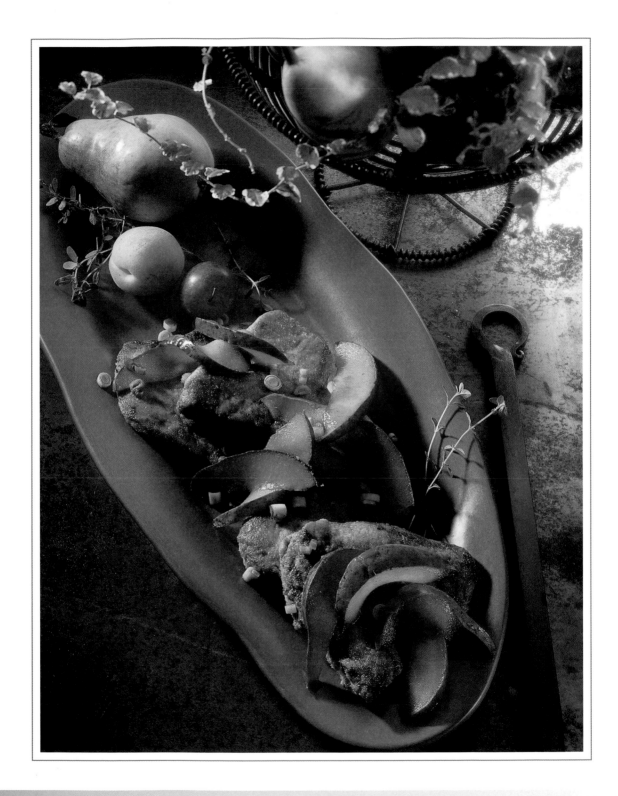

PREPARATION TIME
5 minutes
plus 10 minutes
marinating time

COOKING TIME
20 minutes

Lean Pork Pitas

serves 4

Serving these hot sandwiches with a cool cucumber sauce gives them a Middle Eastern flavor.

8	ounces pork tenderloin
1	tablespoon olive oil
1	tablespoon lemon juice
2	teaspoons Dijon mustard
1	clove garlic, minced
1/2	teaspoon dried oregano
1	cucumber, peeled and diced
1	cup fat-free sour cream
1/2	teaspoon dried dill
1	red onion, thinly sliced
1	green pepper, thinly sliced
4	pita breads, halved
1	cup shredded spinach
8	cherry tomatoes, halved

Cut the pork into 1/2" cutlets, then slice each piece into thin strips.

In a large bowl, mix the oil, lemon juice, mustard, garlic and oregano. Stir in the pork. Cover and refrigerate for 10 minutes or up to 24 hours, turning occasionally.

In a small bowl, mix the cucumbers, sour cream and dill.

In a 9" glass pie plate, mix the onions and peppers. Cover with vented plastic wrap and microwave on high power for 3 minutes, or until soft.

Coat a large no-stick frying pan with no-stick spray and place over medium heat for 2 minutes. Working in batches to avoid overcrowding the pan, add the pork and sauté for 3 minutes, or until cooked through. Transfer to a plate. Add the onions and peppers to the pan; sauté for 3 minutes, or until lightly browned.

Line the pitas with the spinach. Add the pork mixture, tomatoes and cucumber mixture.

Chef's Note
The pork will be easier to slice if you freeze it for about 20 minutes first.

Mustardy Broiled Pork Tenderloins

Serves 4

Serve this German-style pork with sautéed red cabbage.

1	pound pork tenderloin, cut into $3/4$" pieces
2	cloves garlic, minced
$3/4$	cup apple cider
$1/4$	cup honey mustard
1	teaspoon cornstarch

In a resealable plastic bag, mix the pork, garlic, cider and mustard. Shake well. Refrigerate for 30 minutes or up to 24 hours, turning occasionally.

Remove the pork; reserve the marinade. Broil the pork about 4" from the heat for 3 to 5 minutes per side, or until cooked through and no longer pink when tested with a knife.

Pour the marinade into a saucepan and whisk in the cornstarch. Bring to a boil. Cook rapidly until reduced to $1/2$ cup. Serve over the pork.

PER SERVING

204 calories

4.5 g. fat
(20% of calories)

0.2 g. dietary fiber

65 mg. cholesterol

149 mg. sodium

PREPARATION TIME
5 minutes
plus 30 minutes
marinating time

COOKING TIME
10 minutes

Polenta with Italian Sausage, Onions and White Beans

serves 4

PER SERVING

268 calories

4.7 g. fat
(14% of calories)

13 g. dietary fiber

13 mg. cholesterol

688 mg. sodium

A hearty, homey dish for a cold winter night. Who says comfort food can't be healthful?

3½	cups defatted chicken broth
1	cup instant polenta
1	small Italian sausage (2 ounces)
1	small onion, thinly sliced
2	tablespoons orange juice
1	can (19 ounces) cannellini beans
1	teaspoon dried oregano
1	teaspoon fennel seeds
1	teaspoon grated orange rind
2	tablespoons chopped fresh parsley

PREPARATION TIME
10 minutes

COOKING TIME
25 minutes

Bring the broth to a boil in a 2-quart saucepan over high heat. Reduce the heat to low and slowly whisk in the polenta. Cook, stirring occasionally, for 10 minutes, or until very thick.

In a large no-stick frying pan over medium-high heat, cook the sausage for 3 minutes, turning often to brown evenly. Cover and cook for 2 to 3 minutes, or until the sausage is no longer pink when tested with a knife. Slice ½" thick.

Wipe any fat from the pan with a paper towel. Return the pan to the heat, add the onions and sauté for 2 minutes. Add the orange juice; cover and cook for 3 to 4 minutes, or until the onions are very soft. Stir in the beans (with liquid), oregano, fennel seeds, orange rind and sausage.

Spoon the polenta onto a large platter, top with the bean mixture and sprinkle with the parsley.

PREPARATION TIME
10 minutes

COOKING TIME
10 minutes

Lamb Chops
with Cucumbers and Tomatoes

serves 4

Fresh herbs, crisp cucumbers and sweet tomatoes play off the distinctive flavor of quickly seared lamb chops.

1	cup thinly sliced tomatoes
1	cup thinly sliced cucumbers
2	tablespoons orange juice
2	tablespoons chopped fresh mint
1	tablespoon chopped fresh rosemary
1	teaspoon grated orange rind
	Salt and ground black pepper
4	loin lamb chops (about 4 ounces each)

In a medium bowl, mix the tomatoes, cucumbers, orange juice, mint, rosemary and orange rind; add salt and pepper to taste.

Warm a large no-stick frying pan over medium-high heat. Add the lamb and sauté for 5 minutes per side, or until medium-rare. Serve with the tomato mixture.

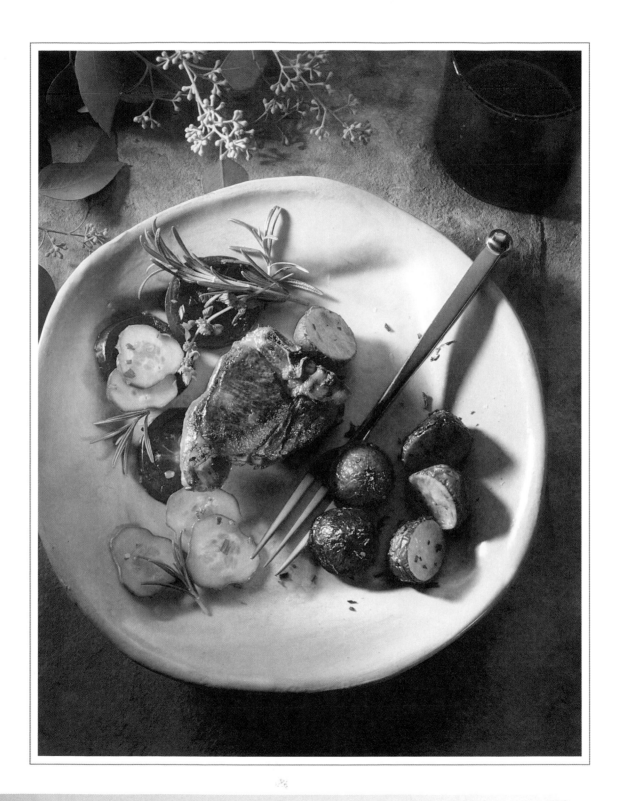

PREPARATION TIME
10 minutes

COOKING TIME
45 minutes

Curried Lamb

serves 8

It tastes exotic but is really easy to make. Serve with a cucumber and yogurt salad.

2	pounds lean leg of lamb, trimmed of all visible fat and cut into $3/4$" cubes
$2\frac{1}{2}$	cups defatted beef broth
$1\frac{1}{2}$	cups chopped onions
1	cup chopped celery
$1\frac{1}{2}$	cups chopped tart apples
2	tablespoons chopped raisins
2	tablespoons curry powder

In a Dutch oven over medium-high heat, brown the lamb in 2 tablespoons of the broth; add more broth if needed.

Add the onions and celery. Cook, stirring, for 2 minutes.

Reduce the heat to medium. Add the apples, raisins, curry powder and the remaining broth. Cover and simmer for 40 minutes, or until the lamb is tender and the sauce is thickened.

Peppered Lamb Loin

serves 4

What a great way to celebrate—or to make even everyday dinner extra special!

PER SERVING

412 calories

11 g. fat
(24% of calories)

1.8 g. dietary fiber

80 mg. cholesterol

150 mg. sodium

1	pound boneless lamb loin, trimmed of all visible fat
2	tablespoons cracked peppercorns
1/4	cup white wine vinegar
1	tablespoon minced shallots
1	cup defatted beef broth
2	tablespoons minced fresh mint
1	tablespoon butter or margarine
8	ounces egg noodles

PREPARATION TIME
10 minutes

COOKING TIME
20 minutes

Cut the lamb into 4 pieces. Firmly press the peppercorns into the cut sides of each piece.

Coat a large no-stick frying pan with no-stick spray and warm over medium-high heat. Add the lamb and sear on both sides. Transfer the lamb to a baking dish and bake at 400° for 10 to 15 minutes, or until cooked through and no longer pink when tested with a knife.

In the same frying pan, mix the vinegar and shallots. Cook over medium heat for 3 minutes, scraping any browned bits from the bottom of the pan. Add the broth, mint and butter or margarine. Bring to a boil; reduce the heat to low.

Cook the noodles in a large pot of boiling water according to the package directions. Drain.

Cut the lamb into very thin slices. Serve over the noodles and drizzle with the mint sauce.

Meatless Meals

VEGETARIAN CASSEROLES, STIR-FRIES AND MORE

No-meat meals have become popular—not only because they're economical but also because they're healthful. Vegetarian dishes bring stimulating variety to our diets through the creative use of vegetables, pasta and dried beans. Meatless meals are power-packed with complex carbohydrates, protein and fiber—and can be very low in fat, calories and cholesterol. Many of this chapter's main dishes are variations of American favorites, such as Eggplant Parmesan and Pasta Primavera, while others are delectable originals, like Curried Chick-Peas and Polenta with Mushroom-Tomato Sauce.

PREPARATION TIME
20 minutes

COOKING TIME
10 minutes

Black Mushroom, Snow Pea and Red Pepper Fricassee

serves 4

Fricassee is generally a dish of stewed or fried meat served in a gravy made from its own juices. Dried shiitake mushrooms replace the meat in this stir-fried vegetarian version.

4	ounces dried shiitake mushrooms
4	scallions, chopped
1	tablespoon chopped fresh ginger
1	clove garlic, minced
2	sweet red peppers, sliced
4	ounces snow peas
1	tablespoon cornstarch
1	cup vegetable broth
2	tablespoons hoisin sauce
1	tablespoon reduced-sodium soy sauce
4	cups cooked couscous

Bring 1 cup water to a boil.

In a small bowl, combine the mushrooms and boiling water. Let stand for 15 minutes. Drain; remove the stems and chop the mushrooms.

Coat a large no-stick frying pan with no-stick spray. Add the scallions, ginger and garlic and cook over medium heat for 1 minute. Add the peppers, snow peas and mushrooms. Cook, stirring, for 3 minutes, or until the vegetables are crisp-tender.

In a small bowl, mix the cornstarch and broth. Add the hoisin sauce and soy sauce. Add to the frying pan and cook for 3 minutes, or until the sauce thickens. Serve over the couscous.

Chef's Note
If shiitake mushrooms are unavailable, substitute 1 ounce dried black mushrooms. Look for both in Asian markets or in the foreign-food aisle of the grocery store.

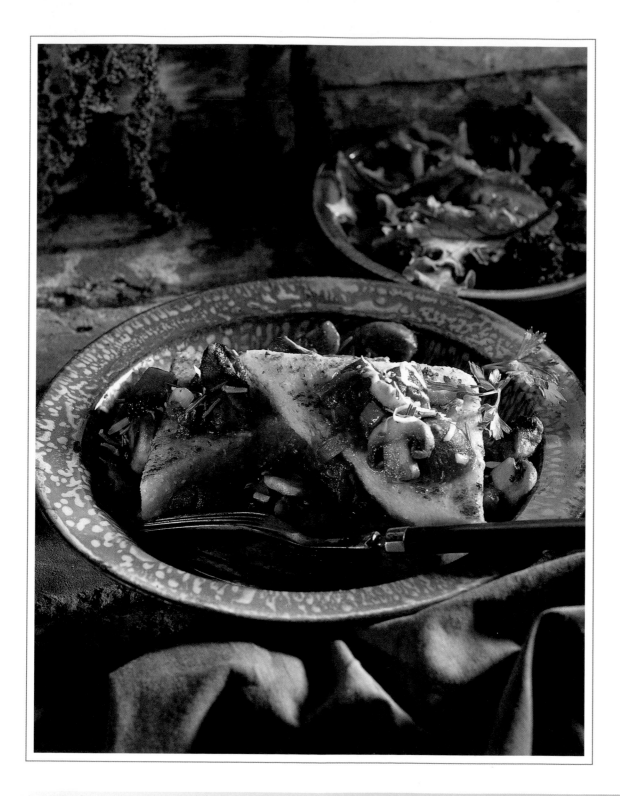

Polenta with Mushroom-Tomato Sauce

serves 4

PER SERVING

214 calories

5.9 g. fat
(24% of calories)

6.2 g. dietary fiber

2 mg. cholesterol

583 mg. sodium

Instant polenta makes this dish fast to prepare.

3½ cups vegetable broth

1   cup instant polenta

2   shallots, minced

2   teaspoons chopped fresh rosemary

1   tablespoon olive oil

4   cups thinly sliced mushrooms

1   cup canned crushed tomatoes

¼   cup white wine or tomato juice

1   tablespoon balsamic vinegar

2   tablespoons grated Parmesan cheese

2   tablespoons chopped fresh parsley

Salt and ground black pepper

PREPARATION TIME
10 minutes

COOKING TIME
30 minutes

Bring the broth to a boil in a 2-quart saucepan over high heat. Reduce the heat to low and slowly whisk in the polenta. Cook, stirring occasionally, for 10 minutes, or until very thick.

In a large no-stick frying pan over medium heat, sauté the shallots and rosemary in the oil for 2 minutes. Stir in the mushrooms, tomatoes, wine or tomato juice and vinegar. Bring to a boil. Cover, reduce the heat and simmer for 5 minutes.

Uncover and cook for 15 to 20 minutes, or until the sauce thickens. Stir in the Parmesan and parsley; add salt and pepper to taste. Serve over the polenta.

Chef's Note

You can easily make this recipe ahead. Pour the cooked polenta into a loaf pan. Cover and refrigerate. To use, cut into 2" slices, place on a baking sheet and bake at 400° for 10 minutes, or until golden brown. Reheat the sauce and serve over the polenta slices.

PREPARATION TIME
5 minutes

COOKING TIME
25 minutes

Curried Chick-Peas

serves 4

*This is curry in a hurry. And unlike so many Indian dishes, it's not loaded
with butter. Serve over rice with warm pitas or Indian flatbread.*

1 1/2	cups vegetable broth
2	cups chopped onions
3	tablespoons grated fresh ginger
1	tablespoon minced garlic
1	sweet red pepper, diced
2	cups cauliflower florets
1	can (16 ounces) chick-peas, rinsed and drained
1–2	tablespoons curry powder
1	teaspoon cornstarch
1/4	cup cold water
	Salt and ground black pepper

Coat a Dutch oven with no-stick spray. Add 1/2 cup of the broth and bring to
a simmer over medium-high heat. Add the onions and cook for 3 minutes.
Add the ginger, garlic, red peppers, cauliflower and chick-peas. Cook for 2
minutes.

Add the remaining 1 cup broth and cook for 5 minutes. Stir in the curry
powder. Cook, stirring occasionally, for 15 minutes, or until the vegetables
are soft.

In a cup, mix the cornstarch and water. Stir into the pot. Cook until the curry
is slightly thickened. Add salt and pepper to taste.

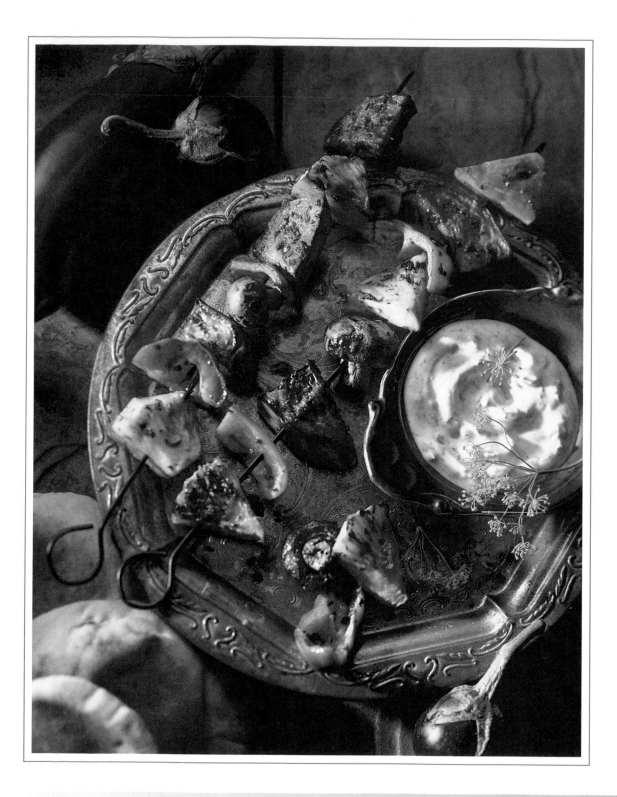

Vegetarian Souvlaki with Pita Wraps

serves 4

PER SERVING

467 calories

6.4 g. fat
(12% of calories)

1.6 g. dietary fiber

1 mg. cholesterol

731 mg. sodium

Consider this Greek fast food. Souvlaki is shish kebab that's generally made with lamb. Here, eggplant and mushrooms give the dish a meaty taste and texture.

PREPARATION TIME
15 minutes
plus 20 minutes
marinating time

COOKING TIME
10 minutes

Souvlaki

½	large eggplant, cubed
12	large button mushrooms
1	green pepper, cubed
6	pineapple rings, quartered
2	tablespoons balsamic vinegar
1	teaspoon dried oregano
2	teaspoons olive oil
1	teaspoon minced garlic
8	large pitas

Tsiziki Dip

1	large cucumber, peeled, seeded, shredded and squeezed dry
1	cup fat-free plain yogurt
1	teaspoon cider vinegar
4	large cloves garlic, minced
1	teaspoon dried dill
	Pinch of salt

In a large bowl, mix the eggplant, mushrooms, peppers, pineapple, vinegar, oregano, oil and garlic. Let stand at room temperature for 20 minutes, stirring frequently.

Thread the vegetables and pineapple onto 8 metal skewers, alternating colors. Grill for 10 minutes, turning once and basting with any leftover marinade.

Warm the pitas on the grill. Wrap a pita around each shish kebab and pull out the skewer.

Meanwhile, in a medium bowl, mix the cucumbers, yogurt, vinegar, garlic, dill and salt. Serve with the souvlaki.

PER SERVING

156 calories

1.5 g. fat
(8% of calories)

3 g. dietary fiber

0 mg. cholesterol

214 mg. sodium

PREPARATION TIME
5 minutes

COOKING TIME
12 minutes

Noodles with Low-Fat Peanut Sauce

serves 4

Try these Asian noodles for a fast and fabulous lunch. Look for udon noodles in the international section of the supermarket.

1	package (9 ounces) Japanese udon noodles
1	tablespoon reduced-sodium soy sauce
2	teaspoons peanut butter
2	teaspoons honey
1	teaspoon minced scallions
1	teaspoon water
$1/2$	teaspoon minced garlic

Cook the noodles in a large pot of boiling water according to the package directions. Drain.

In a large bowl, whisk together the soy sauce, peanut butter, honey, scallions, and water. Add the noodles and toss to mix.

Eggplant Cheese Quesadillas

serves 4

Cheese lovers will eat up these easy tortilla "sandwiches."

PER SERVING

285 calories

7.1 g. fat
(20% of calories)

11.3 g. dietary fiber

25 mg. cholesterol

930 mg. sodium

1	cup diced peeled eggplant
1/2	cup diced tomatoes
1/3	cup chopped scallions
1/4	cup apple juice
1	cup shredded reduced-fat Monterey Jack cheese
1/2	cup fat-free sour cream
1/4	cup grated Parmesan cheese
8	large flour tortillas

PREPARATION TIME
10 minutes

COOKING TIME
20 minutes

In a large no-stick frying pan, combine the eggplant, tomatoes, scallions and apple juice. Cover and cook over medium-high heat for 3 minutes, or until the vegetables are soft. Uncover and cook for 5 minutes, or until the liquid has evaporated.

In a small bowl, combine the Monterey Jack, sour cream and Parmesan. Spread on 4 of the tortillas. Top with the vegetables. Cover with the remaining tortillas.

Wash the frying pan and place over medium heat. Cook each quesadilla for 1 minute per side, or until the cheese melts. Cut into wedges.

PREPARATION TIME
10 minutes

BAKING TIME
15 minutes

Chinese Vegetables in Parchment

serves 4

The flavors of ginger and garlic give these vegetables an extra spark of flavor. Serve the vegetables over noodles.

1   cup sliced onions

1   cup cubed peeled eggplant

2   cups thickly sliced bok choy or Chinese cabbage

1   sweet red pepper, cut into 8 pieces

2   tomatoes, quartered

1   teaspoon minced fresh ginger

1   teaspoon minced garlic

1   cup snow peas

1   cup thickly sliced yellow squash

1   tablespoon rice wine or vegetable broth

$^1/_2$ teaspoon sesame oil

1   tablespoon minced fresh cilantro

Reduced-sodium soy sauce

In a large bowl, mix the onions, eggplant, bok choy or cabbage, peppers, tomatoes, ginger, garlic, snow peas, squash, wine or broth, oil and cilantro.

Tear off 2 large sheets of parchment paper. Divide the vegetables evenly between them and fold to seal. Place on a large baking sheet. Bake at 400° for 15 minutes, or until the vegetables are tender.

Serve the vegetables sprinkled with soy sauce to taste.

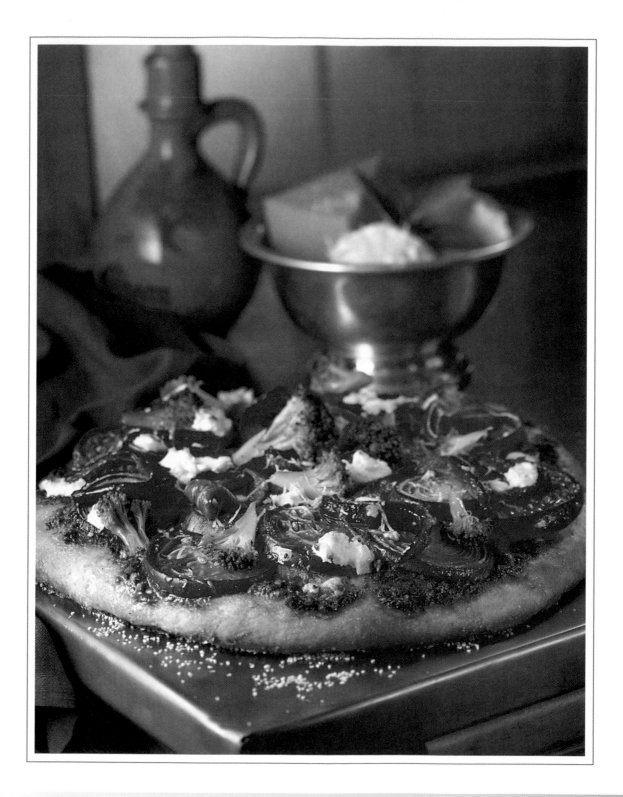

Meatless Meals

Vegetable Pizza with Goat Cheese

serves 4

PER SERVING

375 calories

10.1 g. fat
(24% of calories)

2.9 g. dietary fiber

11 mg. cholesterol

668 mg. sodium

Here's a homemade pie that's in the oven in 10 minutes. The secret is precut vegetables, prepared pizza dough and bought pesto.

1	teaspoon cornmeal
1	pound refrigerated pizza dough
2	tablespoons pesto
1	red onion, thinly sliced
1	large tomato, sliced
1	jar (7 ounces) roasted sweet red peppers, drained
1	cup chopped broccoli florets
1/3	cup crumbled goat cheese
2	tablespoons grated Parmesan cheese

Sprinkle the cornmeal on a pizza pan or large baking sheet. Roll out the dough and place it on the sheet, pressing to fit.

Spread the pesto on the dough; top with the onions and tomatoes. Sprinkle with the peppers, broccoli, goat cheese and Parmesan. Bake at 500° for 10 to 15 minutes, or until the crust is browned and the cheese has melted.

PREPARATION TIME
10 minutes

BAKING TIME
15 minutes

PREPARATION TIME
10 minutes

BAKING TIME
12 minutes

Greengrocer's Pizza

serves 4

Bet you've never had this before. It's a fresh, crispy salad served up in a pizza shell. Popular in trattorias throughout Italy, its success relies on very fresh ingredients.

Crust

1   teaspoon cornmeal

1   pound refrigerated pizza dough

¹/₄ cup shredded provolone cheese

Vegetable Topping

2   tablespoons olive oil

2   teaspoons chopped fresh oregano

1   teaspoon balsamic vinegar

1   teaspoon lemon juice

2   plum tomatoes, cubed

2   tablespoons chopped red onions

2   tablespoons chopped fresh basil

     Salt and ground black pepper

6   cups mixed lettuce

TO MAKE THE CRUST

Sprinkle the cornmeal on a large baking sheet. Divide the dough into 4 pieces and form each into a 6" round. Place on the sheet. Prick the dough deeply all over with a fork.

Bake at 500° for 10 minutes, or until the crusts turn golden brown. Remove from the oven and sprinkle with the provolone. Bake for 2 minutes, or until the provolone melts. Remove the crusts from the oven.

TO MAKE THE VEGETABLE TOPPING

In a large bowl, whisk together the oil, oregano, vinegar and lemon juice. Stir in the tomatoes, onions and basil; add salt and pepper to taste.

Just before serving, add the lettuce to the tomato mixture and toss to coat. Divide the mixture evenly over the crusts.

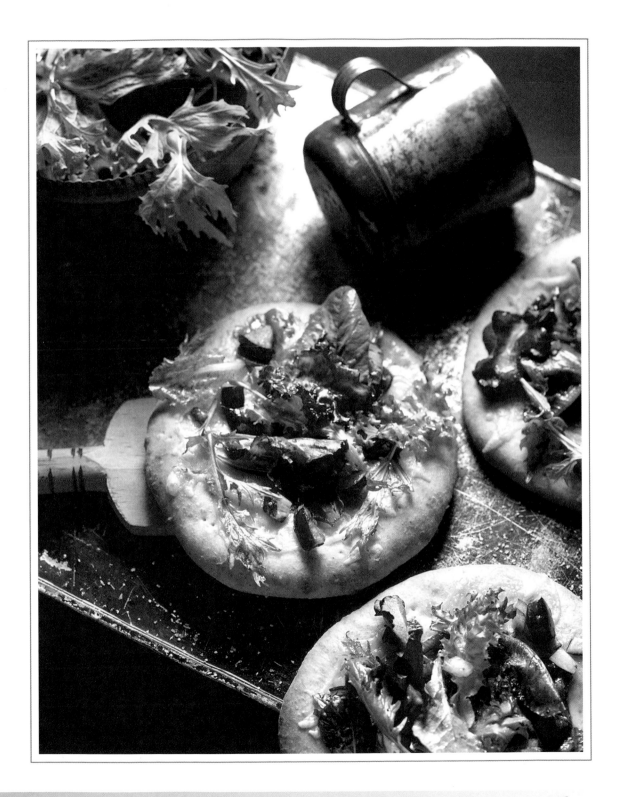

PREPARATION TIME
20 minutes

BAKING TIME
20 minutes

Polenta, Bean and Pasta Casserole

serves 4

You can easily assemble this casserole ahead and bake it at dinnertime.

$\frac{1}{2}$	cup cornmeal
$\frac{1}{2}$	cup cold water
$1\frac{1}{2}$	cups boiling water
$\frac{1}{2}$	cup corn
$\frac{1}{4}$	cup wheat germ
1	green pepper, chopped
4	scallions, chopped
1	teaspoon olive oil
2	ounces Monterey Jack cheese, shredded
4	ounces penne pasta
1	can (16 ounces) kidney beans, rinsed and drained
$1\frac{1}{2}$	cups tomato sauce

In a 2-quart saucepan, whisk together the cornmeal and cold water. Slowly whisk in the boiling water. Bring to a boil over medium heat and cook, stirring constantly, for 10 minutes, or until thick. Stir in the corn and wheat germ.

Coat a 13" × 9" baking dish with no-stick spray. Spread the cornmeal mixture in the dish.

In a large no-stick frying pan over medium heat, sauté the peppers and scallions in the oil for 5 minutes, or until crisp-tender. Spread over the cornmeal. Sprinkle with the Monterey Jack.

Cook the penne in a large pot of boiling water according to the package directions. Drain and return to the pot. Stir in the beans and tomato sauce. Pour over the vegetables.

Cover and bake at 350° for 20 minutes.

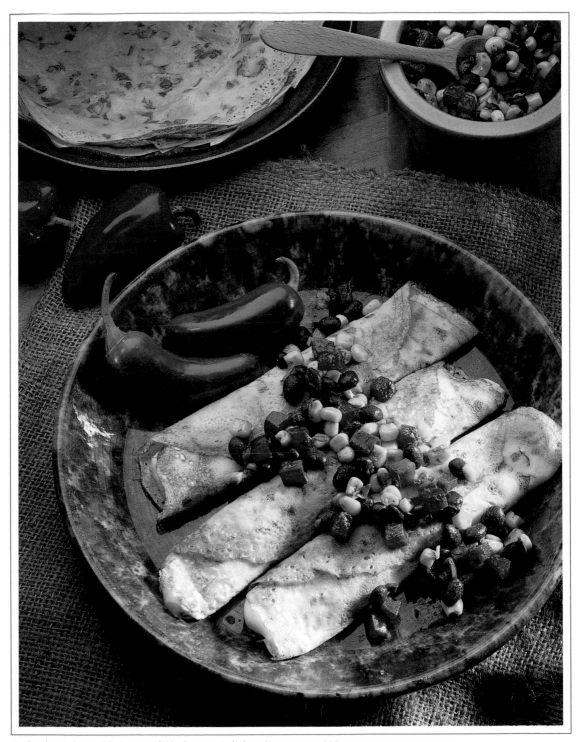

Coriander Crêpes with Corn and Black Bean Relish recipe on page 252

PREPARATION TIME
15 minutes

COOKING TIME
25 minutes

Photo on page 251

Coriander Crêpes with Corn and Black Bean Relish

serves 4

Build a brunch around these zippy crêpes that creatively blend French and Mexican cooking influences. Serve them with pineapple wedges and cornmeal muffins.

Crêpes

1½	cups 1% low-fat milk
1	cup all-purpose flour
½	cup fat-free egg substitute
½	cup chopped fresh coriander
¼	cup chopped scallions

Chili Filling

8	ounces fat-free cream cheese, softened
8	ounces fat-free sour cream
¼	cup chopped green chili peppers
½	teaspoon ground cumin

Corn and Black Bean Relish

1	can (14 ounces) black beans, rinsed and drained
1	can (10 ounces) corn, drained
1	sweet red pepper, diced
2	tablespoons chopped fresh coriander
2	tablespoons lime juice
2	teaspoons olive oil
1	teaspoon chili powder

TO MAKE THE CRÊPES
In a medium bowl, mix the milk, flour, egg substitute, coriander and scallions. The batter should be the consistency of heavy cream; if necessary, thin with a little more milk.

Coat a medium no-stick frying pan with no-stick spray and warm over medium heat. Add about ¼ cup of the batter and swirl to coat the bottom of the pan. Cook the crêpe for 1 minute, or until it easily comes loose from the pan. Turn and cook on the other side for 30 seconds. Transfer to a plate.

Repeat to use all the batter.

TO MAKE THE CHILI FILLING

In a medium bowl, mix the cream cheese, sour cream, peppers and cumin.

TO MAKE THE CORN AND BLACK BEAN RELISH

In a medium bowl, mix the beans, corn, peppers, coriander, lime juice, oil and chili powder.

Place a spoonful of the cream cheese mixture down the middle of each crêpe and roll up. Top with the relish.

Chef's Note

If you use all-purpose flour, let the batter stand for 30 minutes before making the crêpes.

PREPARATION TIME
5 minutes

COOKING TIME
20 minutes

Minted Barley and White Beans

serves 4

Quick-cooking barley lets today's busy cooks use this nutritious old-fashioned grain often.

1	can (15 ounces) cannellini beans, rinsed and drained
1	can (15 ounces) stewed tomatoes, drained
1	cup quick-cooking barley
2	tablespoons chopped fresh mint
1	tablespoon grated lemon rind
2	cups vegetable broth

In a 3-quart saucepan, mix the beans, tomatoes, barley, mint and lemon rind. Stir in the broth. Bring to a boil over high heat. Reduce the heat to medium-low, cover and simmer for 20 minutes, or until the barley is tender and the liquid has been absorbed.

Chick-Pea Fritters with Pepper Sauce

serves 4

Serve these fritters for dinner or even for brunch.

PER SERVING

270 calories

9 g. fat
(30% of calories)

6.6 g. dietary fiber

0 mg. cholesterol

66 mg. sodium

PREPARATION TIME
15 minutes

COOKING TIME
20 minutes

1	jar (7 ounces) roasted sweet red peppers, drained and chopped
1	tomato, diced
1	clove garlic, minced
2	teaspoons balsamic vinegar
1/4	teaspoon honey
1 3/4	cups rinsed and drained canned chick-peas
1	small sweet potato, peeled and finely shredded
1/4	cup finely chopped scallions
1	tablespoon all-purpose flour
2	teaspoons lemon juice
	Pinch of ground black pepper
1/2	cup fat-free egg substitute
2	tablespoons olive oil

In a small bowl, mix the red peppers, tomatoes, garlic, vinegar and honey.

In a medium bowl, coarsely mash the chick-peas with a fork.

In a large bowl, mix the sweet potatoes, scallions, flour, lemon juice and black pepper. Stir in the chick-peas and egg substitute.

Warm 1 tablespoon of the oil in a large no-stick frying pan over medium heat. Drop rounded tablespoonfuls of the chick-pea mixture into the pan, allowing room for them to spread. Cook for 3 minutes per side, or until lightly browned and cooked through. Transfer to a platter and keep warm. Continue making fritters, adding more oil as needed. Serve with the pepper mixture.

PREPARATION TIME
5 minutes

COOKING TIME
10 minutes

Bean and Grain Patties

serves 4

When you're in the mood for burgers but don't want to eat meat, try these inventive look-alikes.

1	can (16 ounces) chick-peas, rinsed and drained
2	eggs
1/3	cup shredded reduced-fat Cheddar cheese
1/4	cup cooked rice
3/4	cup dry bread crumbs
2	tablespoons chopped fresh parsley
3	cloves garlic, minced
2	scallions, chopped
4	pitas
1	tomato, thinly sliced
4	large leaves lettuce
1/2	cup prepared hummus

Using a fork, mash the chick-peas in a medium bowl. Stir in the eggs, Cheddar, rice, bread crumbs, parsley, garlic and scallions.

Coat a large no-stick frying pan with no-stick spray. Using a large spoon, divide the chick-pea mixture into 8 patties (the mixture will be wet); transfer to the frying pan. Cook over medium-high heat for 5 minutes, then turn and flatten with a spatula. Cook for 3 to 5 minutes, or until firm and lightly browned.

Trim one edge off each pita. Open the pitas along the rim and tuck in the patties, tomatoes and lettuce. Top with the hummus.

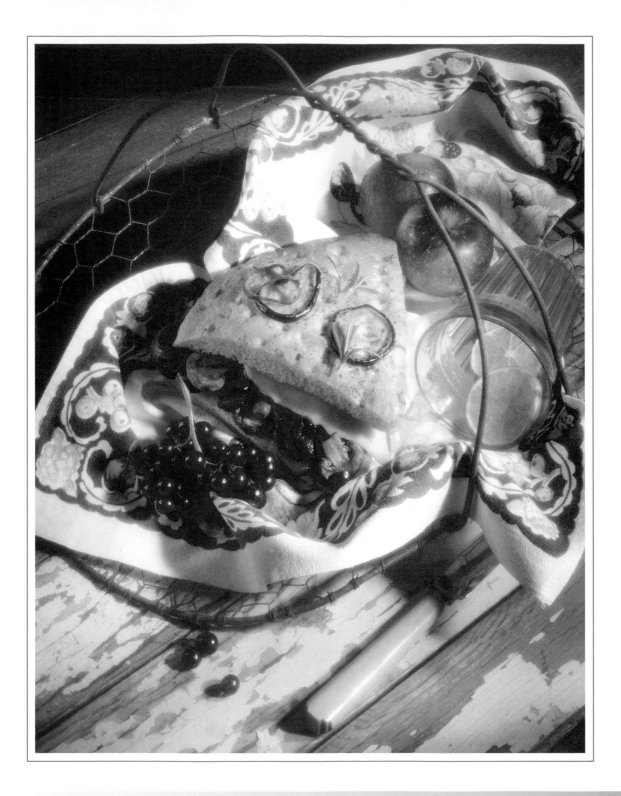

Focaccia with Marinated Vegetables

serves 4

Bright vegetables and mellow cheese are sandwiched in focaccia, which absorbs the flavors of their marinade. This is perfect to take on a hike or a picnic.

PER SERVING

476 calories

16.3 g. fat
(31% of calories)

3.7 g. dietary fiber

5 mg. cholesterol

363 mg. sodium

1 jar (3 1/2 ounces) chopped roasted sweet red peppers, drained

3 cups thickly sliced mushrooms

1 tablespoon pitted and chopped black olives

1 teaspoon drained capers

2 tablespoons balsamic vinegar

1 tablespoon olive oil

1 clove garlic, minced

   Salt and ground black pepper

1 loaf focaccia bread

2 ounces reduced-fat mozzarella cheese, thinly sliced

PREPARATION TIME
10 minutes

In a large bowl, mix the red peppers, mushrooms, olives and capers.

In a cup, whisk together the vinegar, oil and garlic. Pour over the vegetables and toss to coat. Add salt and black pepper to taste.

Cut the focaccia in half horizontally. Cover the bottom half with the vegetable mixture and sprinkle with the mozzarella. Add the top of the focaccia and press firmly. Cut into quarters.

PREPARATION TIME
5 minutes

COOKING TIME
10 minutes

Mediterranean Pasta with Feta and Olives

serves 4

Tangy feta cheese adds surprising richness to this simple pasta dinner without adding a lot of fat.

1	pound penne pasta
2	cups tomato sauce
1/4	teaspoon crushed red-pepper flakes
1 1/2	teaspoons chopped pitted black olives
6	ounces feta cheese, crumbled
1/4	cup chopped fresh parsley

Cook the penne in a large pot of boiling water according to the package directions. Drain and place in a large bowl.

In a 2-quart saucepan, mix the tomato sauce, red-pepper flakes, olives and feta. Cook over medium heat for 3 minutes, or until the feta begins to melt. Stir in the parsley. Pour over the penne and toss to coat.

Meatless Meals

Lemon-Chive Ravioli

serves 4

PER SERVING

189 calories

5.1 g. fat
(24% of calories)

0 g. dietary fiber

24 mg. cholesterol

303 mg. sodium

Ready-made cheese ravioli is available in most markets and cooks in minutes. For an unusual flavor, top it with a lemony white sauce. Serve with breadsticks and a tossed salad.

PREPARATION TIME
5 minutes

COOKING TIME
15 minutes

2	tablespoons all-purpose flour
1½	cups skim milk
1	tablespoon chopped fresh chives
1	teaspoon grated lemon rind
½	teaspoon minced fresh rosemary
4	tablespoons grated Parmesan cheese
9	ounces cheese ravioli

Place the flour in a 2-quart saucepan. Gradually whisk in the milk until smooth. Whisk in the chives, lemon rind, rosemary and 2 tablespoons of the Parmesan. Whisk over medium heat for 5 minutes, or until the mixture comes to a boil and thickens.

Cook the ravioli in a large pot of boiling water according to the package directions. Drain. Serve topped with the sauce and sprinkled with the remaining 2 tablespoons Parmesan.

PREPARATION TIME
5 minutes

COOKING TIME
10 minutes

Pasta Primavera

serves 4

Primavera means "springtime" in Italian. This dish is a medley of fresh spring flavors. You can vary your selection of vegetables with the season.

12	ounces angel hair pasta
3	cloves garlic, minced
1	teaspoon olive oil
1	cup broccoli florets
1/4	cup white wine or vegetable broth
1	sweet red pepper, cut into 1" pieces
1	green pepper, cut into 1" pieces
1	medium zucchini, julienned
1	large carrot, julienned
1/4	cup chopped fresh basil
2	tablespoons shredded Parmesan cheese

Cook the angel hair in a large pot of boiling water according to the package directions. Drain.

In a large no-stick frying pan over medium heat, sauté the garlic in the oil for 1 minute. Add the broccoli and wine or broth; cover and cook for 1 minute.

Add the red peppers, green peppers, zucchini, carrots and basil; cover and cook for 1 minute, or until the vegetables are crisp-tender. Uncover and cook for 1 minute, or until the liquid is reduced. Add the angel hair and toss. Sprinkle with the Parmesan.

Mediterranean Penne

serves 4

Feta cheese and toasted pine nuts give this dish a decidedly Greek flavor.
Use your choice of greens, such as escarole, kale and arugula.

PER SERVING

445 calories

14.4 g. fat
(29% of calories)

7.4 g. dietary fiber

8 mg. cholesterol

169 mg. sodium

PREPARATION TIME
5 minutes

COOKING TIME
15 minutes

10	ounces penne pasta
1	small onion, chopped
2	cloves garlic, minced
1	tablespoon olive oil
4	cups mixed chopped bitter greens
1/4	cup vegetable broth
2	tomatoes, chopped
	Salt and ground black pepper
1/4	cup crumbled feta cheese
1/4	cup toasted pine nuts

Cook the penne in a large pot of boiling water according to the package directions. Drain and place in a large bowl.

In a large no-stick frying pan over medium-high heat, sauté the onions and garlic in the oil for 5 minutes, or until soft. Add the greens and sauté for 1 minute. Add the broth and cook for 1 minute, or until the greens are wilted. Add the tomatoes and salt and pepper to taste.

Toss the greens mixture with the penne. Serve sprinkled with the feta and pine nuts.

PREPARATION TIME
10 minutes

BAKING TIME
30 minutes

Spaghetti with Eggplant and Tomatoes

serves 4

This dish is from Sicily, where abundant eggplant is added to numerous tomato dishes. Often the eggplant is fried; here it is baked to keep fat low.

1	medium eggplant, peeled and cut into $1/2$" slices
1	tablespoon plus 1 teaspoon olive oil
10	ounces spaghetti
$1/2$	cup minced onions
5	cloves garlic, minced
$1 1/2$	pounds plum tomatoes, chopped
$1/4$	cup grated Parmesan cheese
	Salt and ground black pepper
$1/4$	cup chopped fresh basil

Coat a 13" × 9" baking dish with no-stick spray. Add the eggplant. Drizzle with 1 tablespoon of the oil. Cover with aluminum foil and bake at 450° for 25 to 30 minutes, or until tender.

Cook the spaghetti in a large pot of boiling water according to the package directions. Drain.

In a large no-stick frying pan over medium heat, sauté the onions and garlic in the remaining 1 teaspoon oil for 1 minute. Add the tomatoes; cover and cook for 2 minutes, or until soft. Uncover and cook for 2 minutes.

Stir in the eggplant, spaghetti and Parmesan. Add salt and pepper to taste. Toss to mix. Sprinkle with the basil.

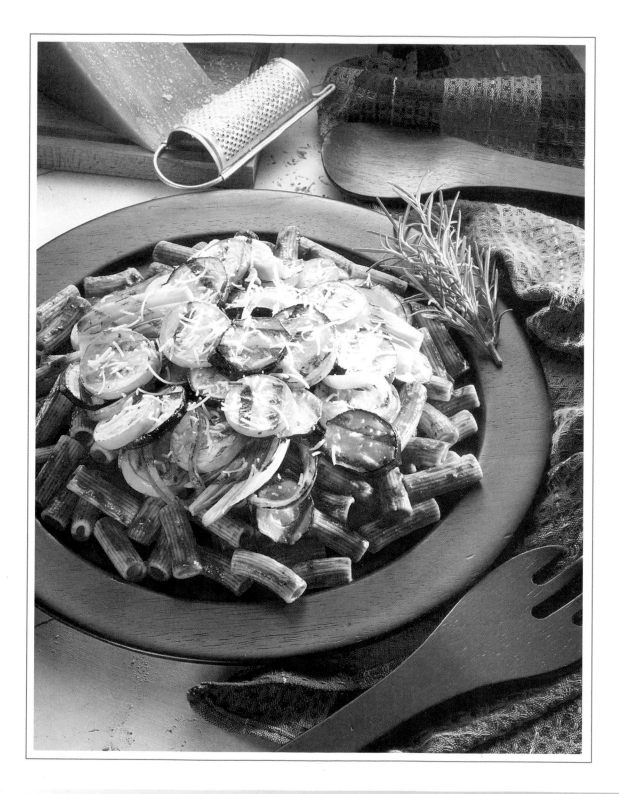

Grilled Vegetable Pasta with Red-Pepper Sauce

serves 4

There's nothing shy or subtle about this color-splashed pasta dish.
Grilling adds a smoky taste to the vegetables, but they also may be broiled.

PER SERVING

95 calories

2.7 g. fat
(23% of calories)

3.4 g. dietary fiber

5 mg. cholesterol

246 mg. sodium

PREPARATION TIME
10 minutes

COOKING TIME
20 minutes

8	ounces rigatoni pasta
2	medium zucchini
2	medium yellow summer squash
2	fennel bulbs, cut into wedges
1	red onion, sliced into ¼" rings
2	tablespoons chopped fresh rosemary
1	jar (7 ounces) roasted sweet red peppers, drained
½	cup vegetable broth
½	teaspoon ground red pepper
¼	cup grated Parmesan cheese

Cook the rigatoni in a large pot of boiling water according to the package directions. Drain and place in a large bowl.

Cut the zucchini and the squash into ¼"-thick diagonal slices. Coat the zucchini, squash, fennel and onions with no-stick spray and sprinkle with the rosemary. Grill for 3 minutes per side, or until golden.

In a blender, process the red peppers, broth and ground red pepper until smooth. Transfer to a 1-quart saucepan and warm over medium heat. Pour over the rigatoni and toss well.

Top with the grilled vegetables and sprinkle with the Parmesan.

PER SERVING

360 calories

6.5 g. fat
(16% of calories)

3.8 g. dietary fiber

79 mg. cholesterol

292 mg. sodium

PREPARATION TIME
10 minutes

COOKING TIME
15 minutes

Lean Fettuccine Alfredo

serves 4

Most recipes for fettuccine Alfredo give you more than a whole day's worth of fat in a single serving. We've kept this recipe nice and light with reduced-fat dairy products.

8	ounces fettuccine
1/2	cup fat-free cottage cheese
1/4	cup evaporated skim milk
1/4	cup reduced-fat ricotta cheese
1/4	cup shredded reduced-fat Monterey Jack cheese
1/4	cup grated Parmesan cheese
1	teaspoon minced garlic
2	tablespoons minced parsley

Cook the fettuccine in a large pot of boiling water according to the package directions. Drain.

In a blender or food processor, process the cottage cheese, milk and ricotta until smooth. Transfer to a large no-stick frying pan and add the Monterey Jack, Parmesan and garlic. Stir over medium heat for 3 to 5 minutes, or until the cheeses are melted and the sauce is smooth.

Add the fettuccine and toss to coat. Heat through. Sprinkle with the parsley.

30-Minute Manicotti

serves 4

Who'd believe real Italian manicotti could be this quick? Part of the secret is cooking the assembled dish in the microwave.

PER SERVING

332 calories

6.8 g. fat
(19% of calories)

2.1 g. dietary fiber

74 mg. cholesterol

568 mg. sodium

8	manicotti shells
2	cups reduced-fat ricotta cheese
1	cup finely chopped spinach
1	egg
1/4	cup grated Parmesan cheese
2	tablespoons minced fresh basil
1/4	cup chopped fresh parsley
1/4	teaspoon ground nutmeg
2	cups tomato sauce
1 1/2	cups shredded fat-free mozzarella cheese

PREPARATION TIME
15 minutes

COOKING TIME
15 minutes

Cook the manicotti in a large pot of boiling water according to the package directions. Drain and transfer to a bowl of cold water.

In a medium bowl, mix the ricotta, spinach, egg, Parmesan, basil, parsley and nutmeg. Drain the manicotti shells and fill each with about 1/4 cup of the mixture.

Spoon 1 cup of the tomato sauce into an 11" × 7" microwave-safe baking dish. Arrange the shells in the pan; spoon the remaining 1 cup tomato sauce on top. Sprinkle with the mozzarella. Cover with vented plastic wrap.

Microwave on medium-high (70% power) for 15 minutes, or until the sauce is bubbly; rotate the dish every 5 minutes during cooking.

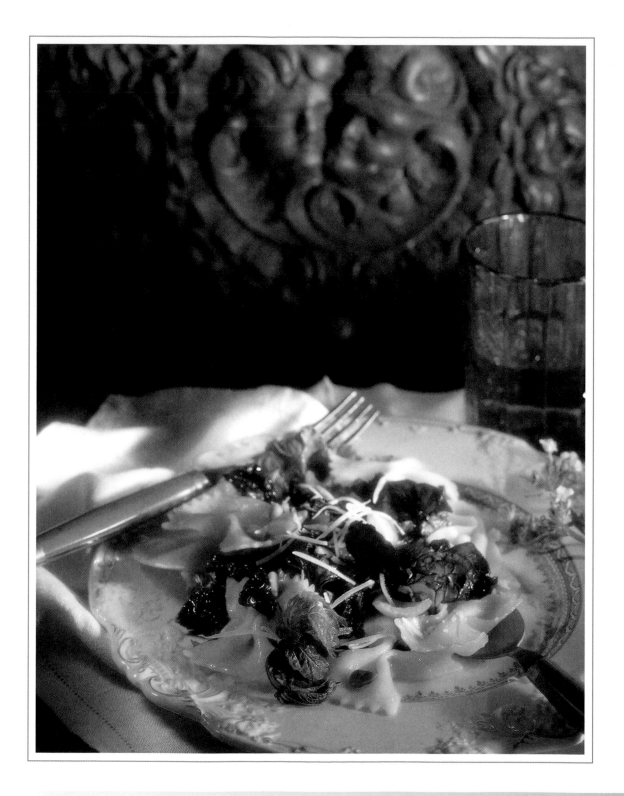

Farfalle with Braised Bitter Greens

serves 4

Farfalle is also known as butterflies or bow ties. Use a combination of bitter greens such as beet greens, collards, kale, mustard greens, broccoli rabe and turnip greens in this quick pasta dish.

PER SERVING

380 calories

12.4 g. fat
(29% of calories)

2 g. dietary fiber

68 mg. cholesterol

186 mg. sodium

¼	cup chopped sun-dried tomatoes
½	cup boiling water
10	ounces farfalle pasta
1	small onion, chopped
2	cloves garlic, minced
1	tablespoon olive oil
4	cups mixed bitter greens, coarsely shredded
¼	cup vegetable broth
3	dashes of hot-pepper sauce
	Salt and ground black pepper
¼	cup shredded Asiago or other sharp cheese
¼	cup toasted pine nuts

PREPARATION TIME
5 minutes

COOKING TIME
15 minutes

In a small bowl, combine the tomatoes and water.

Cook the farfalle in a large pot of boiling water according to the package directions. Drain and place in a large bowl.

In a large frying pan over medium-high heat, sauté the onions and garlic in the oil for 4 minutes. Add the greens and sauté for 1 minute. Add the broth and cook for 1 minute, or until the greens are wilted. Drain the tomatoes and add to the pan. Add the hot-pepper sauce and salt and pepper to taste.

Toss the greens with the pasta. Sprinkle with the cheese and pine nuts.

chapter 9

Classic Accompaniments

ALL-TIME FAVORITE SIDE DISHES

Think of a meal's main dish as the star and the side dishes as the supporting cast. They make the star look (and in this case, taste) great, but they can also earn some applause on their own. Side dishes enhance the entrée by providing contrasting or complementary flavors, colors and textures. They also bolster the healthful benefit of a meal by adding nutrients that the main dish lacks. Here are classic accompaniments that are easy to prepare and will complement everything from meat loaf to grilled salmon steaks.

Classic Accompaniments

Cheesy Twice-Baked Potatoes

serves 4

Everybody loves twice-baked potatoes. And you'll feel good about serving them when they're this low in fat.

4	medium russet potatoes
2	tablespoons minced onions
3	tablespoons fat-free sour cream
1	tablespoon chopped fresh parsley
	Pinch of ground black pepper
1	tablespoon shredded reduced-fat Cheddar cheese
1/4	teaspoon paprika

Pierce the potatoes in several places with a fork and microwave on high power for 7 to 10 minutes, turning once, or until the potatoes are tender. Let stand for 5 minutes, or until cool enough to handle.

Coat a small no-stick frying pan with no-stick spray and warm over medium heat. Add the onions and sauté for 3 to 4 minutes, or until lightly browned.

Slice 1/4" off the top of each potato and scoop out the center with a spoon, leaving a 1/4"-thick shell. Place the centers in a medium bowl and mash with a fork. Stir in the onions, sour cream, parsley and pepper.

Spoon the filling into the potato shells and top with the Cheddar. Sprinkle with the paprika.

Place the potatoes on a baking sheet and bake at 475° for 3 to 5 minutes, or until the filling is hot and the Cheddar has melted.

PER SERVING

134 calories

0.4 g. fat
(3% of calories)

1.6 g. dietary fiber

0 mg. cholesterol

47 mg. sodium

PREPARATION TIME
20 minutes

BAKING TIME
5 minutes

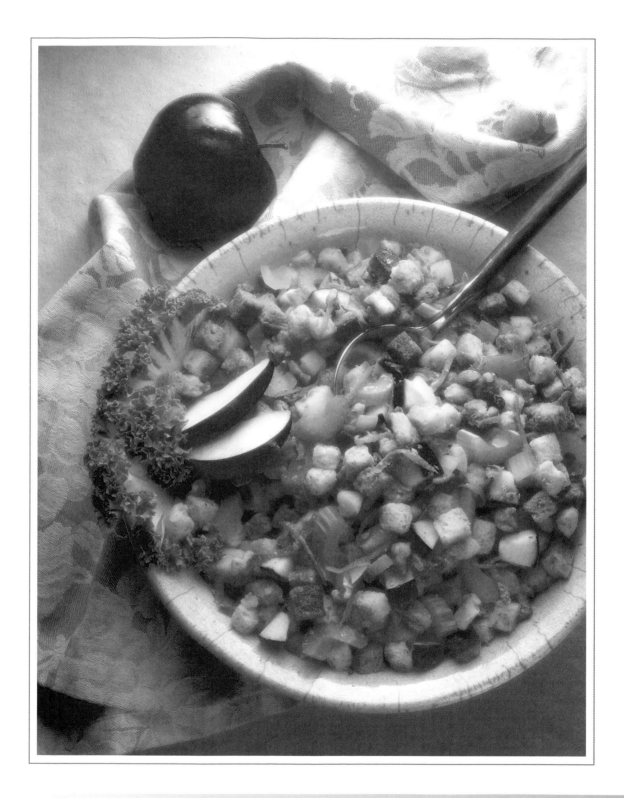

Classic Accompaniments

Apple-Walnut Stuffing

serves 8

If you love stuffing but hate the large serving of fat you get with most types, try this lighter version. Serve as an accompaniment to roast poultry or even simple sautéed chicken breasts.

PER SERVING

225 calories

11 g. fat
(44% of calories)

3.2 g. dietary fiber

0 mg. cholesterol

198 mg. sodium

PREPARATION TIME
15 minutes

BAKING TIME
45 minutes

2	onions, chopped
4	stalks celery, sliced
1	medium carrot, shredded
1	tablespoon olive oil
1¼	cups defatted chicken broth
¼	cup fat-free egg substitute
2	medium apples, chopped
½	cup walnuts, coarsely chopped
3	tablespoons chopped fresh parsley
1	teaspoon dried rosemary
¼	teaspoon ground black pepper
6½	cups bread cubes

In a 3-quart saucepan over medium-high heat, sauté the onions, celery and carrots in the oil for 5 minutes, or until soft. Remove from the heat. Stir in the broth, egg substitute, apples, walnuts, parsley, rosemary and pepper. Add the bread cubes and mix well.

Coat a 13" × 9" baking dish with no-stick spray. Add the stuffing. Cover with aluminum foil and bake at 325° for 45 minutes, or until browned.

PREPARATION TIME
5 minutes

COOKING TIME
10 minutes

Celebration Rice

serves 4

Any occasion will be cause for celebration if you serve this festive dish.

1¼	cups quick-cooking brown rice
1	cup water
⅓	cup orange juice
1	tablespoon reduced-sodium soy sauce
1½	teaspoons olive oil
1	teaspoon grated orange rind
1	teaspoon curry powder
1	tablespoon toasted sesame seeds
2	tablespoons chopped fresh chives
2	tablespoons diced sweet red peppers

In a 2-quart saucepan over medium-high heat, bring the rice, water, orange juice, soy sauce, oil, orange rind and curry powder to a boil. Cover, reduce the heat to medium-low and simmer for 10 minutes, or until all the liquid has been absorbed.

Fluff the rice with a fork. Stir in the sesame seeds, chives and peppers.

Barley Pilaf

serves 4

This satisfying side dish uses quick-cooking barley, which is ready in a fraction of the time needed for regular pearl barley. Serve the pilaf with sautéed chicken breasts or pork tenderloin cutlets.

PER SERVING

170 calories

2.7 g. fat
(13% of calories)

5.4 g. dietary fiber

0 mg. cholesterol

52 mg. sodium

PREPARATION TIME
5 minutes

COOKING TIME
20 minutes

2	cups defatted chicken broth
1	cup quick–cooking barley
1	bay leaf
1	cup diced carrots
1	onion, diced
¼	cup sliced scallions
1	clove garlic, minced
1	teaspoon olive oil

In a 2-quart saucepan over medium-high heat, bring the broth, barley and bay leaf to a boil. Cover and cook over medium-low heat for 15 minutes, or until the barley is tender and the liquid has been absorbed. Remove and discard the bay leaf. Fluff the barley with a fork.

In a large no-stick frying pan over medium heat, sauté the carrots, onions, scallions and garlic in the oil for 5 minutes, or until the vegetables are just tender. Add the barley and toss to combine.

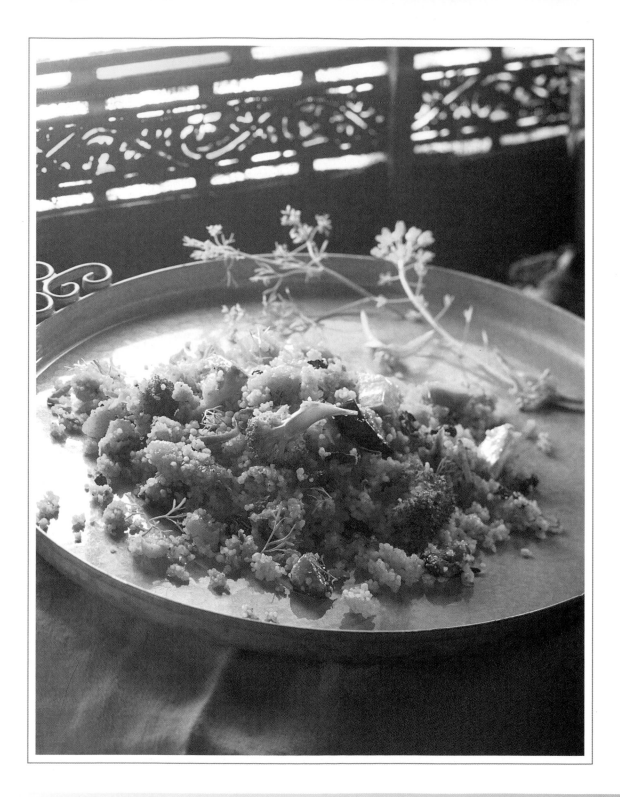

Classic Accompaniments

East Indian Curried Couscous

serves 8

This elegant side dish blends Middle Eastern and Indian ingredients. Serve it in place of rice as an accompaniment to fish or chicken.

PER SERVING

222 calories

1.1 g. fat
(4% of calories)

8.8 g. dietary fiber

0 mg. cholesterol

76 mg. sodium

PREPARATION TIME
10 minutes

COOKING TIME
10 minutes

1/2	cup sliced scallions
1/2	cup shredded carrots
1	cup broccoli florets
1	teaspoon olive oil
1/4	cup currants
1/4	cup chopped dried apricots
2	cups couscous
1 1/2	cups defatted chicken broth
1	cup apple juice
1–2	teaspoons curry powder
1	cup chopped yellow summer squash
1/2	cup diced tomatoes
	Salt and ground black pepper
1/4	cup chopped fresh cilantro or mint

In a large no-stick frying pan over medium-high heat, sauté the scallions, carrots and broccoli in the oil for 5 minutes, or until the vegetables are tender. Stir in the currants, apricots, couscous, broth, apple juice and curry powder. Bring to a boil.

Stir in the squash and tomatoes. Cover and remove from the heat. Let stand for 5 minutes, or until all the liquid has been absorbed. Fluff with a fork and add salt and pepper to taste. Sprinkle with the cilantro or mint.

PREPARATION TIME
10 minutes

COOKING TIME
15 minutes

Wild Rice Pancakes

serves 4

Wild rice is actually a type of grass, not a true rice. These quick pancakes are good served with a dollop of fat-free sour cream and snipped chives or with applesauce.

$1/4$	cup fat-free egg substitute
1	tablespoon all-purpose flour
1	tablespoon skim milk
$1/4$	teaspoon baking powder
$1/8$	teaspoon dried thyme
$1/8$	teaspoon ground black pepper
1	cup cooked wild rice
3	tablespoons minced onions
2	tablespoons chopped fresh parsley

In a medium bowl, whisk together the egg substitute, flour, milk, baking powder, thyme and pepper. Stir in the wild rice, onions and parsley.

Coat a large no-stick frying pan with no-stick spray and warm over medium heat for 2 minutes. Working in batches, drop tablespoons of the mixture onto the pan and press down to flatten. Cook for 1 to 2 minutes per side, or until firm and lightly browned.

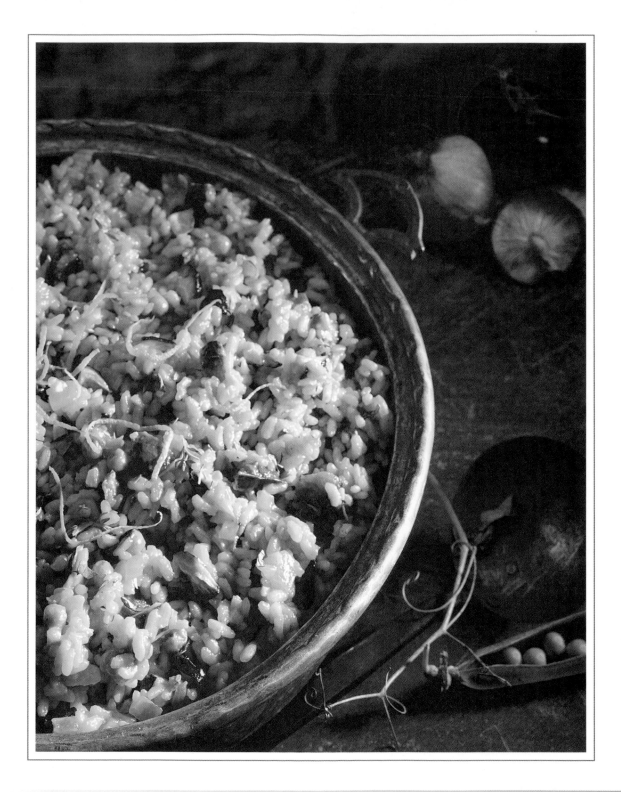

Saffron Risotto with Vegetables

serves 8

Saffron is the yellow-orange stigmas of a small purple crocus and is the world's most expensive spice. Fortunately, a little of this spice goes a long way. In this dish, the saffron turns the rice into a lovely golden backdrop for the bright peas and tomatoes.

PER SERVING

130 calories

2 g. fat
(14% of calories)

0.4 g. dietary fiber

0 mg. cholesterol

188 mg. sodium

PREPARATION TIME
10 minutes

COOKING TIME
30 minutes

1	cup Arborio rice (see note)
1/2	cup finely chopped onions
1/2	cup finely chopped shiitake mushrooms
1	tablespoon olive oil
2	cloves garlic, minced
1	teaspoon Dijon mustard
1/2	teaspoon crushed saffron threads
1/8	teaspoon ground nutmeg
	Pinch of ground cloves
1/4	cup orange juice
1	teaspoon grated orange rind
3	cups defatted chicken broth
1/4	cup peas
1	plum tomato, diced
1	teaspoon chopped fresh thyme
2	tablespoons chopped fresh basil
	Salt and ground black pepper

In a large microwave-safe bowl, mix the rice, onions, mushrooms, oil, garlic, mustard, saffron, nutmeg and cloves. Microwave on high power for 2 minutes.

Stir in the orange juice, orange rind and 2 cups of the broth. Microwave for 10 minutes, stirring after 5 minutes. Stir in the remaining 1 cup broth. Microwave for 15 minutes, stirring after 7 minutes.

Stir in the peas, tomatoes and thyme. Microwave for 1 minute. Stir in the basil. Add salt and pepper to taste.

Chef's Note
Arborio rice is a short-grain variety from Italy that produces creamier dishes than regular long-grain rice. It's available in most large supermarkets.

Garlic Mashed Potatoes

serves 4

PER SERVING

145 calories

0.2 g. fat
(1% of calories)

1.5 g. dietary fiber

0 mg. cholesterol

38 mg. sodium

PREPARATION TIME
5 minutes

COOKING TIME
15 minutes

Photo on page 144

There's virtually no fat in these wonderfully creamy potatoes. We've eliminated the fat by replacing the usual butter and heavy cream with fat-free sour cream and skim milk.

4	medium potatoes, peeled and cubed
6	cloves garlic
$1/3$	cup skim milk
$1/4$	cup fat-free sour cream

Place the potatoes and garlic in a 3-quart saucepan and add cold water to cover. Bring to a boil over high heat. Reduce the heat to medium and cook for 15 minutes, or until the potatoes are tender.

Drain well and return the mixture to the pan. Off heat, mash with a potato masher until smooth. Add the milk and stir over medium heat for 1 minute. Stir in the sour cream.

Spicy Vegetable Pot Pies with Johnny Cake Crust

serves 4

Pioneers called the cornmeal bread they made on a griddle johnny cakes. In this recipe, cornmeal crusts top individual vegetable casseroles. We've used buttermilk and egg substitute to reduce the fat.

PER SERVING

210 calories

3.2 g. fat
(13% of calories)

4.8 g. dietary fiber

1.1 mg. cholesterol

486 mg. sodium

PREPARATION TIME
20 minutes

BAKING TIME
20 minutes

Vegetable Filling

1	cup chopped zucchini
1	cup chopped carrots
1	cup chopped onions
1/2	cup water
1 1/2	cups salsa

Johnny Cake Crust

1/2	cup cornmeal
1/2	cup all-purpose flour
1	teaspoon baking powder
1/2	cup low-fat buttermilk
1/4	cup fat-free egg substitute
1	tablespoon honey

TO MAKE THE VEGETABLE FILLING
In a large no-stick frying pan over medium heat, cook the zucchini, carrots, onions and water for 5 minutes, or until the vegetables are just tender. Add the salsa and cook for 5 minutes.

Divide among 4 individual casserole dishes.

TO MAKE THE JOHNNY CAKE CRUST
In a medium bowl, mix the cornmeal, flour and baking powder.

In a small bowl, mix the buttermilk, egg substitute and honey. Pour over the flour mixture and stir until blended.

Spoon the crust mixture over the vegetables. Bake at 350° for 20 minutes, or until the top is brown and the vegetables are bubbling.

PREPARATION TIME
10 minutes

COOKING TIME
35 minutes

Shallot and Corn Risotto

serves 8

Creamy risotto is the ultimate comfort food. Here, we've enhanced it with corn and sweet red peppers. This side dish could also be a main course for four.

3½	cups defatted chicken broth
3	tablespoons minced shallots
1	teaspoon olive oil
¼	cup dry sherry or water
2	tablespoons minced sweet red peppers
1	cup Arborio rice
2	cups cooked corn
1	tablespoon minced fresh parsley
	Salt and ground black pepper

Bring the broth to a simmer in a 1-quart saucepan over medium heat. Reduce the heat to low and keep the broth warm.

In a 2-quart saucepan over medium-high heat, cook the shallots in the oil for 2 minutes. Add the sherry or water, red peppers and ¼ cup of the broth; cook for 3 minutes.

Add the rice and stir for 1 minute. Add ½ cup of the remaining broth. Stirring continuously, cook until the liquid has completely evaporated. Continue to add broth in ½-cup increments until the rice is creamy and just tender (about 25 minutes total time).

Stir in the corn and parsley. Add salt and pepper to taste.

Chef's Note
For a creamier risotto, puree 1 cup of the corn.

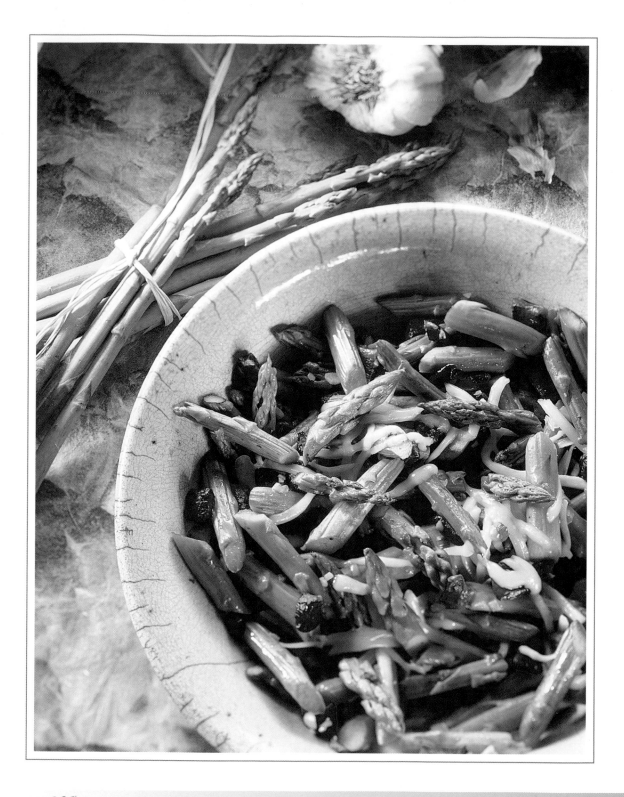

Asparagus with Roasted Peppers and Olives

serves 4

PER SERVING

52 calories

1.8 g. fat
(27% of calories)

0.4 g. dietary fiber

4 mg. cholesterol

43 mg. sodium

A lively dish that's wonderful alongside grilled or broiled pork or chicken. Tossed with pasta, it becomes a light meal. It is equally good hot or at room temperature.

PREPARATION TIME
5 minutes

COOKING TIME
5 minutes

1	pound asparagus, cut into 1" pieces
2	cloves garlic, minced
2	tablespoons lemon juice
1	jar (3½ ounces) chopped roasted sweet red peppers, drained
2	tablespoons chopped pitted black olives
1	tablespoon chopped fresh parsley
	Dash of hot-pepper sauce
	Salt and ground black pepper
2	tablespoons shredded provolone cheese

Coat a large no-stick frying pan with no-stick spray. Add the asparagus and garlic; stir over medium-high heat for 1 minute. Add the lemon juice. Cover and cook for 2 minutes, or until the asparagus is bright green and crisp-tender.

Stir in the red peppers, olives, parsley and hot-pepper sauce. Add salt and black pepper to taste. Sprinkle with the provolone.

PREPARATION TIME
15 minutes

COOKING TIME
11 minutes

Marinated Vegetables

serves 8

You can make this dish a day or two ahead so the vegetables absorb the marinade and the flavors have time to blend. Serve chilled or at room temperature.

Marinade

1/2	cup white wine vinegar
1	tablespoon olive oil
1	teaspoon lemon juice
1	teaspoon Dijon mustard
1	teaspoon sugar
1	clove garlic, minced
2	tablespoons chopped fresh marjoram
2	tablespoons chopped fresh parsley

Vegetables

8	ounces new potatoes, cubed
1	cup broccoli florets
1	sweet red pepper, cut into 2" pieces
1	cup quartered mushrooms
1/2	cup sliced scallions
2	tablespoons sliced pitted black olives
	Salt and ground black pepper

TO MAKE THE MARINADE
In a large bowl, whisk together the vinegar, oil, lemon juice, mustard, sugar and garlic. Stir in the marjoram and parsley,

TO MAKE THE VEGETABLES
In a large microwave-safe dish, microwave the potatoes on high power for 8 minutes, or until tender. Add to the marinade while still hot.

In the same microwave-safe dish, microwave the broccoli for 3 minutes, or until crisp-tender. Add to the marinade. Stir in the peppers, mushrooms, scallions and olives. Add salt and black pepper to taste.

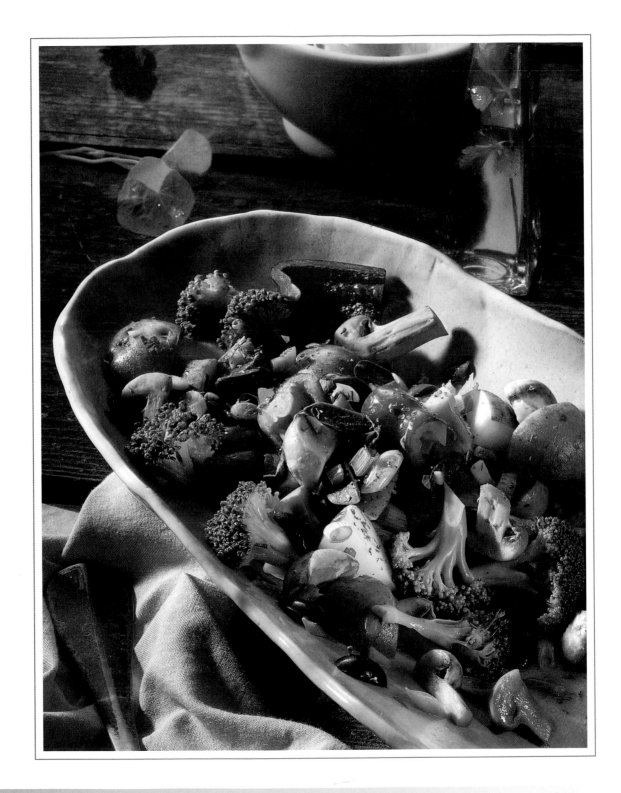

Spicy Corn on the Cob

serves 4

PER SERVING

155 calories

4.3 g. fat
(22% of calories)

2.7 g. dietary fiber

0 mg. cholesterol

6 mg. sodium

PREPARATION TIME
5 minutes

COOKING TIME
20 minutes

Photo on page 120

Prepare this corn anytime you're having a cookout. It can grill in its own foil packet while your main dish is cooking.

4	ears corn, shucked
2	tablespoons balsamic vinegar
1	tablespoon olive oil
¼	teaspoon ground red pepper

Place the corn on a large sheet of aluminum foil.

In a small bowl, stir together the vinegar, oil and pepper. Brush on the corn. Seal the foil tightly. Grill for 20 minutes, or until the corn is cooked through; turn the packet after 10 minutes.

Oven-Fried Pepper-Dusted Potato Wedges

Serves 4

PER SERVING

220 calories

0.2 g. fat
(1% of calories)

2.2 g. dietary fiber

0 mg. cholesterol

16 mg. sodium

PREPARATION TIME
10 minutes

COOKING TIME
20 minutes

Photo on page 213

They're wonderful steak fries, but they're virtually fat-free since they aren't deep-fried.

4	medium russet potatoes
	Ground red pepper
	Salt and ground black pepper

Pierce the potatoes in several places with a fork and microwave on high power for 7 to 10 minutes, turning once, or until the potatoes are tender. Let stand for 5 minutes, or until cool enough to handle.

Cut each potato into 8 wedges and place on a baking sheet. Mist with no-stick spray and lightly sprinkle with the red pepper, salt and black pepper. Bake at 475° for 20 minutes, or until the potatoes are crisp and brown.

Balsamic Broccoli Rabe

serves 4

PER SERVING

45 calories

0.9 g. fat
(15% of calories)

3.1 g. dietary fiber

1 mg. cholesterol

59 mg. sodium

Broccoli rabe is a green vegetable that has long stalks and scattered clusters of buds that resemble broccoli flowers. It has a pungent flavor that has made it a favorite in Italy for many years. It has become widely available in groceries here.

1	pound broccoli rabe
1	tablespoon balsamic vinegar
1	tablespoon grated Parmesan cheese
2	teaspoons butter-flavored sprinkles
1	teaspoon minced fresh thyme

PREPARATION TIME
5 minutes

COOKING TIME
5 minutes

Rinse the broccoli rabe in cold water and shake off excess water. Cut the thick stems into 1" pieces; cut the leafy tops into 3" pieces. Place in a Dutch oven with just the water left clinging to the pieces.

Cover and cook over medium heat for 5 minutes, or until tender. Drain. Sprinkle with the vinegar, Parmesan, butter-flavored sprinkles and thyme. Toss to mix.

Classic Accompaniments

Roasted Peppers in Marinade

serves 4

Roasting sweetens bell peppers and gives them a hint of smokiness. Serve them with grilled or sautéed chicken, pork or fish. Or add them to pasta, green salads, risotto or polenta.

PER SERVING

20 calories

0.1 g. fat
(4% of calories)

0.9 g. dietary fiber

0 mg. cholesterol

2 mg. sodium

PREPARATION TIME
5 minutes

COOKING TIME
15 minutes

1	large sweet red pepper
1	large yellow pepper
1	large orange pepper
2	tablespoons chopped fresh basil
1	tablespoon balsamic vinegar
1	clove garlic, minced

Place the peppers on a large baking sheet and broil about 5" from the heat until blackened on all sides. Wrap in damp paper towels and allow to stand for 5 minutes, or until cool enough to handle. Remove the skin, seeds and veins. Slice the peppers into ½" strips and place in a medium bowl. Add the basil, vinegar and garlic; toss to mix.

PREPARATION TIME
5 minutes

COOKING TIME
15 minutes

Garlicky Green Beans

serves 4

Don't be concerned about the amount of garlic used here. Boiling mellows and sweetens its distinctive flavor.

6	cloves garlic
1	pound green beans
2	tablespoons lemon juice
1	teaspoon olive oil
$\frac{1}{8}$	teaspoon ground black pepper

Bring a large pot of water to a boil over medium-high heat. Add the garlic and cook for 10 minutes, or until the garlic is tender when pierced with the tip of a knife. Remove with a slotted spoon and place in a small bowl.

Add the beans to the water. Cook for 5 minutes, or until the beans are crisp-tender. Drain and return the beans to the pot.

Mash the garlic with a fork. Stir in the lemon juice, oil and pepper. Pour over the beans and toss to coat.

Chef's Note

To easily remove the skin from a clove of garlic, cut the root end off and firmly press the flat side of a wide knife blade on the clove. The skin will loosen and the clove will easily slip out. This same technique can be used to ease mincing once the clove is peeled.

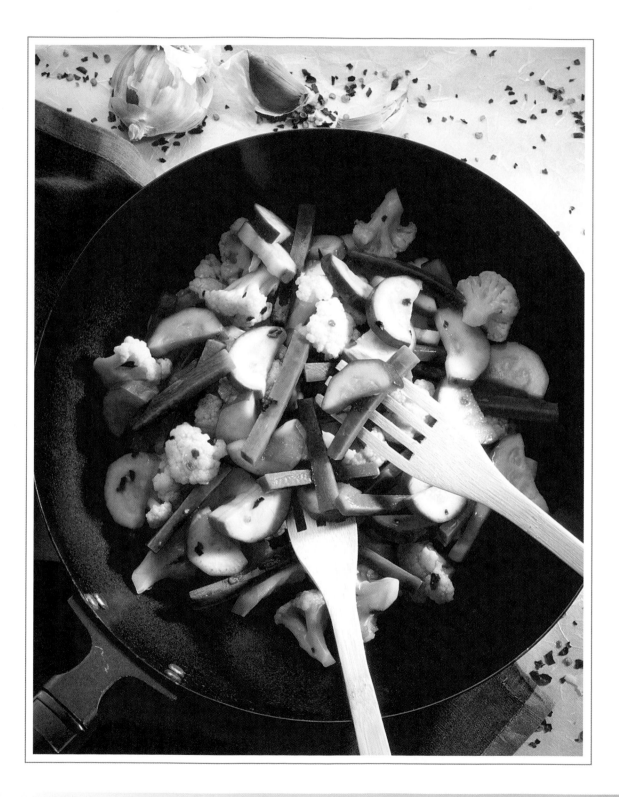

Classic Accompaniments

Asian Vegetable Sauté

Serves 4

These vegetables take only minutes to prepare and make a flavorful accompaniment to flank steak or pork tenderloin.

PER SERVING

176 calories

4.2 g. fat
(20% of calories)

6 g. dietary fiber

0 mg. cholesterol

599 mg. sodium

2	cups cauliflower florets
1	carrot, julienned
2	teaspoons olive oil
1	zucchini, halved lengthwise and thinly sliced
1/4	cup defatted chicken broth
1	teaspoon sesame oil
2	tablespoons reduced-sodium soy sauce
1	teaspoon grated fresh ginger
1	teaspoon cornstarch
1/2	teaspoon red-pepper flakes

PREPARATION TIME
10 minutes

COOKING TIME
5 minutes

In a large no-stick frying pan over medium-high heat, stir-fry the cauliflower and carrots in the olive oil for 2 minutes. Add the zucchini and stir-fry for 2 minutes.

In a small bowl, mix the broth, sesame oil, soy sauce, ginger, cornstarch and red-pepper flakes. Add to the pan. Stir for 1 minute, or until the sauce thickens.

PREPARATION TIME
10 minutes

COOKING TIME
20 minutes

Golden Mashed Potatoes with Horseradish

serves 4

Classic recipes for mashed potatoes call for lots of butter. But you can get a rich flavor by replacing the butter with cottage cheese. And to get the golden color that butter-drenched potatoes have, use yellow-fleshed spuds such as Yellow Finnish, Yukon Golds or Yellow Golds.

$1\frac{1}{2}$	pounds yellow-fleshed potatoes, peeled and cubed
1	cup 1% low-fat milk
$1\frac{1}{2}$	cups reduced-fat cottage cheese
4	scallions, minced
1	tablespoon prepared horseradish
$\frac{1}{2}$	teaspoon ground black pepper
	Pinch of ground nutmeg

Place the potatoes in a 3-quart saucepan and add cold water to cover. Bring to a boil over high heat. Reduce the heat to medium and cook for 15 minutes, or until the potatoes are tender.

Drain well and return the potatoes to the pan. Off heat, mash with a potato masher until smooth. Add the milk and stir over medium heat for 1 minute.

In a food processor, process the cottage cheese until smooth. Stir into the potatoes. Stir in the scallions, horseradish, pepper and nutmeg.

Baked Radicchio

serves 4

PER SERVING

44 calories

1.2 g. fat
(24% of calories)

2.1 g. dietary fiber

0 mg. cholesterol

37 mg. sodium

*Radicchio's distinctive bite is as bright as its beautiful magenta leaves.
Here, the flavor is tempered by baking. This makes a marvelous companion
to roast chicken or sautéed chicken breasts.*

1	pound radicchio
¾	cup diced carrots
¾	cup diced celery
½	cup chopped onions
¼	cup minced shallots
¼	cup water
	Salt and ground black pepper
1	teaspoon olive oil

PREPARATION TIME
10 minutes

BAKING TIME
40 minutes

Trim and clean the radicchio. Cut into quarters and remove the core.

In an 11" × 7" baking dish, mix the carrots, celery, onions, shallots and water. Lay the radicchio on top of the vegetables. Add salt and pepper to taste. Cover tightly with aluminum foil.

Bake at 400° for 15 minutes. Reduce the heat to 350° and bake for 25 minutes, or until the radicchio is tender. Sprinkle with the oil.

PREPARATION TIME
5 minutes

COOKING TIME
25 minutes

Molasses Baked Beans

serves 4

Baked beans are an all-American dish. To create a lighter version, we used reduced-fat turkey sausage rather than bacon. Although they're cooked on top of the stove to save time, these beans retain their baked-all-day flavor.

$^{1}/_{3}$	cup reduced-fat turkey sausage
$^{3}/_{4}$	cup diced onions
1	can ($14^{1}/_{2}$ ounces) pinto beans, rinsed and drained
$^{1}/_{4}$	cup molasses
3	tablespoons chili sauce
2	teaspoons Worcestershire sauce

Crumble the sausage into a 2-quart saucepan. Cook over medium heat for 3 minutes, breaking up the sausage with a wooden spoon. Add the onions and cook for 3 to 4 minutes, or until the onions are translucent.

Stir in the beans, molasses, chili sauce and Worcestershire sauce. Bring to a boil, reduce the heat to medium-low and cook for 10 to 15 minutes, or until the sauce has thickened.

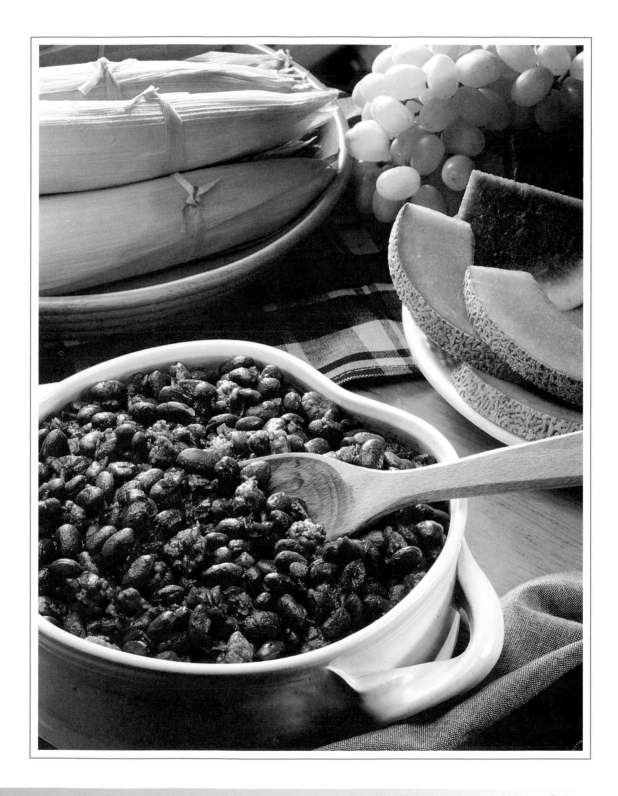

PREPARATION TIME
3 minutes

COOKING TIME
15 minutes

Photo on page 214

Honey-Glazed Carrots

Serves 4

Give ordinary carrots extraordinary flavor with this sweet-tart glaze. They're a great accompaniment to most any meat or poultry main course.

1   cup orange juice

1   pound baby carrots

1   tablespoon balsamic vinegar

1   tablespoon honey

Bring the orange juice to a boil in a large no-stick frying pan over medium-high heat. Add the carrots. Reduce the heat to medium, cover and cook for 10 minutes, or until the carrots are tender. Stir in the vinegar and honey. Stir over medium-high heat for 3 minutes, or until most of the liquid has evaporated and the carrots are lightly glazed.

PREPARATION TIME
5 minutes

BAKING TIME
30 minutes

Corn Pudding

serves 4

This old-fashioned soufflé has its roots in New England and is a classic accompaniment for roasts, wild game, lobster or clams.

1   package (10 ounces) frozen corn, thawed

1   cup fat-free egg substitute

$1/4$ cup all-purpose flour

3   tablespoons maple syrup

In a blender, combine the corn, egg substitute, flour and maple syrup. Blend on high speed for 20 to 25 seconds, or until the corn is finely chopped.

Coat a 1-quart casserole with no-stick spray. Add the corn mixture. Bake at 425° for 25 to 30 minutes, or until slightly puffed and a knife inserted into the center comes out clean.

Maple Pecan Squash

serves 4

PER SERVING

136 calories

2.5 g. fat
(15% of calories)

1.6 g. dietary fiber

0 mg. cholesterol

21 mg. sodium

Maple syrup is a luscious, fat-free way to add flavor to squash. Any other winter squash would also work well in this recipe.

1	medium butternut squash, peeled and shredded
1/3	cup maple syrup
1/8	teaspoon ground black pepper
1/4	cup fresh bread crumbs
2	tablespoons chopped pecans

In a medium bowl, mix the squash, maple syrup and pepper.

Coat a 1½-quart casserole with no-stick spray. Add the squash mixture and sprinkle with the bread crumbs and pecans. Bake at 425° for 20 to 25 minutes, or until the squash is tender.

PREPARATION TIME
10 minutes

BAKING TIME
25 minutes

Baked Goodies

FRESH FROM THE OVEN OR GRIDDLE

Wake up to a breakfast of crisp waffles, dress up a main dish with a round focaccia bread piping hot from the oven or make an open-faced sandwich on a slice of home-baked bread. You can enjoy these goodies, even as you pare fat from your diet. Ingredients such as skim milk, buttermilk and fat-free sour cream greatly reduce the fat without compromising the flavor of these baked treats. We've adapted a whole bakery full of tempting favorites such as pound cake, coffee cake, pandowdy and muffins to fit your lower-fat lifestyle.

Baked Goodies

Country-Style Blueberry Muffins

makes 12

These streusel-topped muffins have a tender crumb with minimal fat.

PER MUFFIN

147 calories

2.9 g. fat
(17% of calories)

1.2 g. dietary fiber

21 mg. cholesterol

186 mg. sodium

2   tablespoons + 1 1/2 cups all-purpose flour

2   tablespoons packed brown sugar

1/2 teaspoon ground cinnamon

1   tablespoon cold butter or margarine, cut into small pieces

1/2 cup sugar

2   teaspoons baking powder

1/2 teaspoon salt

1/2 cup skim milk

3   tablespoons fat-free vanilla yogurt

1   egg

1   tablespoon canola oil

1   teaspoon vanilla

1/2 teaspoon grated lemon rind

1 1/2 cups blueberries

PREPARATION TIME
10 minutes

BAKING TIME
20 minutes

In a small bowl, mix 2 tablespoons of the flour, brown sugar, and cinnamon. With 2 knives, cut in the butter or margarine until the mixture resembles coarse meal. Set aside.

Preheat the oven to 400°. Coat a 12-cup muffin pan with no-stick spray.

In a large bowl, whisk together the remaining 1 1/2 cups flour, sugar, baking powder, and salt.

In a medium bowl, whisk together the milk, yogurt, egg, oil, vanilla and lemon rind. Pour over the flour mixture and stir just until combined; do not overmix. Gently stir in the blueberries.

Divide the batter evenly among the muffins cups, filling them two-thirds full. Sprinkle each muffin with 1 teaspoon of the topping.

Bake for 17 to 20 minutes, or until a toothpick inserted in the center of a muffin comes out clean. Cool on a wire rack for 5 minutes before removing from the pan.

PREPARATION TIME
15 minutes

BAKING TIME
25 minutes

Bran Muffins

makes 12

*Most bran muffins are high in fat, despite their reputation as a health food.
In our version, skim milk and egg whites keep the muffins light, while whole-
wheat flour and bran cereal give them a hearty texture and delicious flavor.*

½	cup all-purpose flour
½	cup whole-wheat flour
1	tablespoon baking powder
¼	teaspoon salt
¼	teaspoon ground cinnamon
1	cup skim milk
2	tablespoons canola oil
2	tablespoons honey
3	egg whites
1	cup All-Bran cereal

Preheat the oven to 400°. Coat a 12-cup muffin pan with no-stick spray.

In a large bowl, whisk together the all-purpose flour, whole-wheat flour,
baking powder, salt and cinnamon.

In a medium bowl, whisk together the milk, oil, honey and egg whites. Stir in
the cereal and let stand for 10 minutes. Pour over the flour mixture and stir
just until combined; do not overmix.

Divide the batter evenly among the muffin cups, filling them two-thirds full.

Bake for 20 to 25 minutes, or until a toothpick inserted in the center of a
muffin comes out clean. Cool on a wire rack for 5 minutes before removing
from the pan.

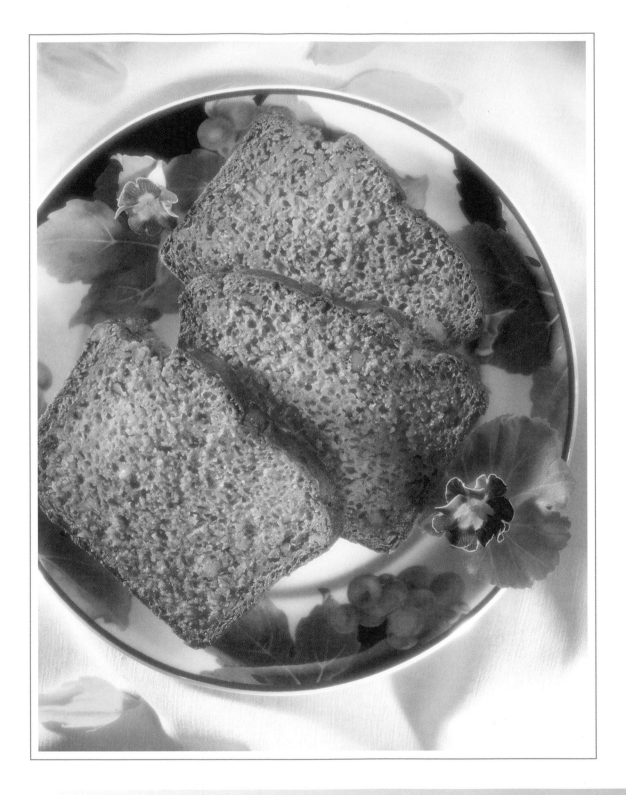

Baked Goodies

Spiced Pumpkin Bread

makes 1 loaf; 18 slices

A mixture of spices gives this quick bread real pumpkin pie flavor.

PER SLICE

91 calories

1.6 g. fat
(15% of calories)

0.7 g. dietary fiber

12 mg. cholesterol

92 mg. sodium

PREPARATION TIME
10 minutes

BAKING TIME
45 minutes

1½	cups all-purpose flour
2	tablespoons cornstarch
¾	teaspoon baking powder
½	teaspoon baking soda
¼	teaspoon salt
⅛	teaspoon ground allspice
⅛	teaspoon ground cloves
¼	teaspoon ground cinnamon
¼	teaspoon ground nutmeg
1	egg
1	egg white
⅓	cup sugar
¼	cup packed brown sugar
1	cup canned pumpkin
6	tablespoons low-fat buttermilk
1½	tablespoons canola oil
½	teaspoon vanilla

Preheat the oven to 350°. Coat a 9" × 5" loaf pan with no-stick spray.

In a large bowl, whisk together the flour, cornstarch, baking powder, baking soda, salt, allspice, cloves, cinnamon and nutmeg.

In a medium bowl, whisk together the egg, egg white, sugar and brown sugar until smooth. Whisk in the pumpkin, buttermilk, oil and vanilla. Pour over the flour mixture and stir just until combined; do not overmix.

Spoon the batter into the pan. Bake for 45 minutes, or until a toothpick inserted in the center comes out clean. Cool on a wire rack for 10 minutes. Remove from the pan and cool completely.

PREPARATION TIME
10 minutes

BAKING TIME
25 minutes

Maple Banana Bake

serves 4

This warm treat takes only 10 minutes to assemble. Pop it in the oven to bake while you enjoy dinner.

4	bananas, peeled and diagonally sliced
1/4	cup maple syrup
1	teaspoon lime juice
1/2	cup rolled oats
1/4	cup all-purpose flour
2	tablespoons apple juice
1	teaspoon melted butter
1/2	teaspoon vanilla
	Pinch of ground nutmeg
	Pinch of ground cinnamon
1/4	cup reduced-fat sour cream
2	tablespoons packed brown sugar

Preheat the oven to 400°. Lightly oil a shallow casserole dish.

Spread the bananas evenly in the dish. Drizzle with the maple syrup and lime juice.

In a small bowl, mix the oats, flour, apple juice, butter, vanilla, nutmeg and cinnamon. Sprinkle over the bananas.

Bake for 25 minutes, or until the topping is crisp.

In a cup, mix the sour cream and brown sugar. Serve over the bananas.

Apple Apricot Pandowdy

serves 4

PER SERVING

308 calories

2.6 g. fat
(8% of calories)

5.1 g. dietary fiber

0 mg. cholesterol

944 mg. sodium

A biscuit crust tops this deep-dish fruit dessert. To serve, break up the crust with a spoon or knife and stir it into the filling.

2	Golden Delicious apples, peeled and sliced
1/2	cup water
1/4	cup chopped dried apricots
1/4	cup frozen apple juice concentrate, thawed
1	tablespoon molasses
3/4	cup reduced-fat baking mix
1/3	cup skim milk
1/4	teaspoon ground cinnamon

PREPARATION TIME
10 minutes

COOKING TIME
15 minutes

In a large no-stick frying pan over medium heat, cook the apples, water, apricots, apple juice concentrate and molasses for 5 minutes, or until the apples soften.

In a medium bowl, mix the baking mix, milk and cinnamon with a fork until just blended. Drop by spoonfuls on top of the apple mixture.

Cover and cook for 10 minutes, or until the crust is cooked through. Serve warm.

PREPARATION TIME
10 minutes

BAKING TIME
55 minutes

Cornmeal Blueberry Cake

makes 1 loaf; 8 slices

Here's a dense, lemony loaf cake with a light texture.

1 1/2	cups all-purpose flour
1/2	cup cornmeal
1 1/2	teaspoons baking powder
1/2	teaspoon salt
1/4	teaspoon baking soda
2/3	cup fat-free plain yogurt
1	tablespoon lemon juice
1	teaspoon vanilla
3/4	cup sugar
1/4	cup oil
2	teaspoons grated lemon rind
1	egg
1	egg white
1	cup blueberries

Preheat the oven to 350°. Coat an 8" × 4" loaf pan with no-stick spray.

In a small bowl, whisk together the flour, cornmeal, baking powder, salt and baking soda.

In another small bowl, whisk together the yogurt, lemon juice and vanilla.

In a medium bowl, stir together the sugar, oil and lemon rind. Beat in the egg and egg white. Alternately beat in the flour mixture and the yogurt mixture, beginning and ending with the flour mixture. Mix just until combined; do not overmix. Gently stir in the blueberries.

Pour the batter into the pan. Bake for 45 to 55 minutes, or until a toothpick inserted in the center comes out clean. Cool on a wire rack for 10 minutes. Remove from the pan and cool completely.

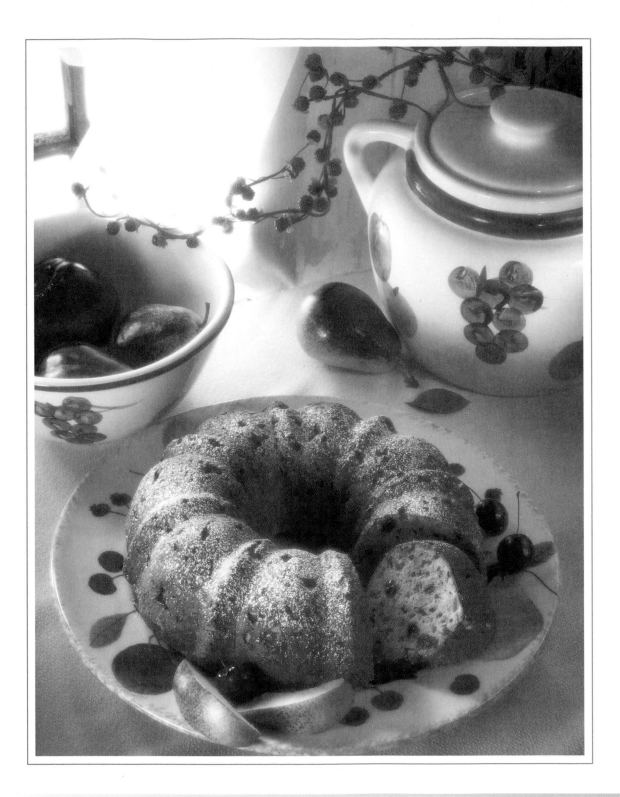

Pecan Coffee Cake

serves 9

Egg substitute and fat-free sour cream are the keys to keeping this coffee cake light. If desired, sprinkle the batter with streusel topping (see Country-Style Blueberry Muffins, page 319) before baking.

1 1/2	cups all-purpose flour
2	teaspoons baking powder
1/2	teaspoon baking soda
1/2	teaspoon salt
1/4	teaspoon ground cinnamon
1/2	cup packed brown sugar
2	tablespoons butter or margarine, softened
3/4	cup fat-free egg substitute
1/2	cup fat-free sour cream
1	cup raisins
1/2	cup chopped pecans

PREPARATION TIME
10 minutes

BAKING TIME
40 minutes

Preheat the oven to 350°. Coat an 8" Bundt pan with no-stick spray.

In a medium bowl, whisk together the flour, baking powder, baking soda, salt and cinnamon.

In a large bowl, beat together the brown sugar and butter or margarine until smooth. Beat in the egg substitute and sour cream.

Gradually beat in the flour mixture until the batter is smooth. Stir in the raisins and pecans.

Spread the batter evenly in the baking dish. Bake for 35 to 40 minutes, or until a toothpick inserted in the center comes out clean. Cool for 10 minutes on a wire rack. Remove and cool completely.

PREPARATION TIME
10 minutes

Pineapple Pound Cake

serves 8

Instant pudding and store-bought pound cake make this a quick treat when unexpected company arrives.

1	package (1 ounce) sugar-free vanilla instant pudding mix
1½	cups skim milk
½	teaspoon almond extract
1	can (20 ounces) crushed pineapple in juice
¼	cup chopped toasted almonds
1	fat-free pound cake (12 ounces)
	Mandarin orange slices or sliced strawberries

Place the pudding mix in a large bowl; add the milk and almond extract. Whisk for 2 minutes. Let stand for 5 minutes to thicken.

Place the pineapple in a strainer and press with the back of a spoon to remove as much of the juice as possible; reserve the juice for another use. Fold the pineapple and almonds into the pudding.

Cut the cake into 8 slices. Spoon the pudding mixture over the slices. Top with the oranges or strawberries.

Chef's Note

For a more elegant presentation, cut the cake horizontally into 3 layers. Place 1 layer, cut side up, on a serving platter. Spread with one-third of the pudding mixture. Repeat twice to use all the cake and pudding. Decorate with the oranges or strawberries. If the layers slide while the pudding is still soft, hold them in place by spearing the cake with skewers at the corners. Chill before serving.

Orange Poppyseed Loaf

makes 1 loaf; 18 slices

Orange extract and orange yogurt put a new twist on a popular poppyseed brunch or breakfast bread.

2	cups all-purpose flour
1⅓	cups whole-wheat flour
3	tablespoons poppyseeds
4	teaspoons baking soda
1	cup fat-free orange yogurt
¼	cup canola oil
¼	cup honey
1	tablespoon orange extract

Preheat the oven to 350°. Coat a 9" × 5" loaf pan with no-stick spray.

In a large bowl, whisk together the all-purpose flour, whole-wheat flour, poppyseeds and baking soda.

In a medium bowl, whisk together the yogurt, oil, honey and orange extract. Pour over the flour mixture and mix until the dough forms a rough-looking mass.

Place on a lightly floured surface and knead until the dough comes together. Using your hands, roll the dough into a log shape (the dough will be sticky). Press the dough into the pan, being sure to press it firmly into the corners.

Bake for 30 to 35 minutes, or until a toothpick inserted in the center comes out clean. Cool on a wire rack for 10 minutes. Remove from the pan and cool completely.

PER SLICE

142 calories

4 g. fat
(25% of calories)

1.5 g. dietary fiber

0 mg. cholesterol

191 mg. sodium

PREPARATION TIME
10 minutes

BAKING TIME
35 minutes

PREPARATION TIME
15 minutes

COOKING TIME
20 minutes

Strawberry Waffles
with Strawberry-Rhubarb Sauce

serves 4

The Dutch are given credit for introducing waffles to this country in 1796. These have a double dose of strawberries from preserves and frozen berries. During the summer, use a pint of fresh berries.

Strawberry Waffles

1 1/4	cups all-purpose flour
1	teaspoon baking soda
1	cup low-fat buttermilk
1/4	cup all-fruit strawberry spread
2	tablespoons fat-free egg substitute
2	tablespoons canola oil
1	egg white

Strawberry-Rhubarb Sauce

1	package (10 ounces) frozen strawberries, thawed
1	cup sliced rhubarb
2	tablespoons honey
1	tablespoon grated orange rind

TO MAKE THE STRAWBERRY WAFFLES

Preheat a waffle iron according to the manufacturer's directions.

In a medium bowl, whisk together the flour and baking soda.

In a small bowl, whisk together the buttermilk, fruit spread, egg substitute and oil. Pour over the flour mixture and mix well.

In another small bowl, beat the egg white with a clean whisk until soft peaks form. Fold into the batter.

Use about 1/2 cup of the batter per waffle and bake according to the manufacturer's directions.

TO MAKE THE STRAWBERRY-RHUBARB SAUCE

In a 2-quart saucepan over medium heat, cook the strawberries, rhubarb, honey and orange rind for 5 minutes, or until the rhubarb is tender. Serve warm or at room temperature.

PREPARATION TIME
10 minutes

COOKING TIME
15 minutes

Raspberry Bread Pudding

serves 8

*Here's an excellent way to use up stale bread. For variety, you may replace
the raspberries with blueberries, pitted cherries or chopped peaches. You may
also use other types of bread, such as whole-grain or raisin.*

1 1/2	cups skim milk
3/4	cup fat-free egg substitute
1/2	cup honey
1	teaspoon vanilla
1/4	teaspoon ground cinnamon
1/4	teaspoon ground nutmeg
4	cups oat bread cubes
2	cups raspberries

In a large bowl, whisk together the milk, egg substitute, honey, vanilla,
cinnamon and nutmeg. Stir in the bread and raspberries.

Coat a 2-quart casserole dish with no-stick spray. Add the bread mixture.
Cover with a lid or vented plastic wrap. Microwave on medium (50% power)
for 14 minutes, stirring the mixture every 3 minutes.

Chocolate Crêpes with Berries

serves 4

PER SERVING

266 calories

3.2 g. fat
(10% of calories)

2 g. dietary fiber

109 mg. cholesterol

124 mg. sodium

Along the streets of Paris, you'll find walk-up crêpe stands where Parisians buy crêpes-to-go filled with sugar, chocolate, jam, cheese or ham. Serve this elegant fruit-filled version at a brunch, shower or summertime tea.

PREPARATION TIME
5 minutes

COOKING TIME
15 minutes

½	cup all-purpose flour
2	tablespoons unsweetened cocoa powder
½	cup skim milk
2	eggs
2	tablespoons honey
2	cups fat-free frozen vanilla yogurt
2	cups fresh berries

In a medium bowl, whisk together the flour and cocoa powder. Whisk in the milk, eggs and honey. The batter should be the consistency of heavy cream; if necessary, thin with a little more milk.

Coat a medium no-stick frying pan with no-stick spray. Warm over medium heat. Add about 3 tablespoons of the batter and swirl to coat the bottom of the pan. Cook the crêpe for 1 minute, or until it easily comes loose from the pan. Turn and cook the other side for 30 seconds. Transfer to a plate.

Repeat to use all the batter.

To serve, place a small scoop of the frozen yogurt on each crêpe and roll to enclose the filling. Sprinkle with the berries.

Chef's Note

If you use all-purpose flour, let the batter stand for 30 minutes before cooking the crêpes.

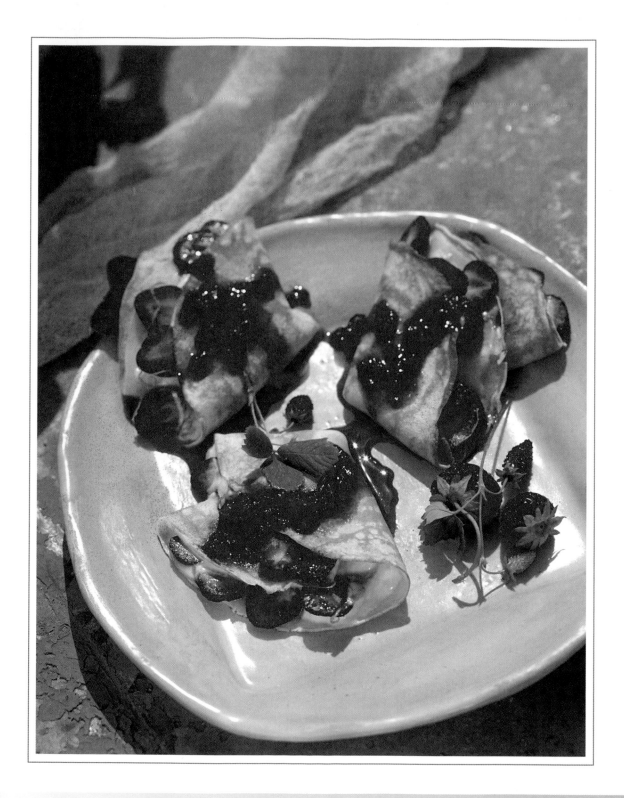

Strawberry Crêpes

serves 4

PER SERVING

249 calories

4.1 g. fat
(15% of calories)

2 g. dietary fiber

23 mg. cholesterol

381 mg. sodium

A lot lower in fat than traditional strawberry shortcake, these crêpes have all the same elegance and flavor. Look for prepared crêpes in the produce section of your supermarket or use the ones in Chocolate Crêpes with Berries (page 335). This easy dessert is great during strawberry season.

PREPARATION TIME
10 minutes

4	ounces fat-free cream cheese
1	cup fat-free sour cream
1/4	cup packed brown sugar
1	teaspoon grated orange rind
1/2	teaspoon vanilla
8	crêpes
3	cups sliced strawberries
1	tablespoon honey

In a food processor, process the cream cheese, sour cream, brown sugar, orange rind, and vanilla until smooth. Divide among the crêpes and sprinkle with 2 cups of the strawberries. Roll up the crêpes.

In a food processor, puree the remaining 1 cup strawberries with the honey. Drizzle over the crêpes.

PREPARATION TIME
5 minutes

COOKING TIME
20 minutes

Whole-Grain Corn Waffles

serves 8

Serve these luscious waffles with warmed maple syrup and fresh berries or all-fruit preserves.

1 1/2	cups whole-wheat flour
1/2	cup cornmeal
2	cups low-fat buttermilk
2	tablespoons canola oil
2	eggs
1	egg white
1	tablespoon packed brown sugar
1/4	teaspoon salt
1/2	cup corn

Preheat a waffle iron according to the manufacturer's directions.

In a blender, process the flour, cornmeal, buttermilk, oil, eggs, egg white, brown sugar, and salt until smooth. Pour into a medium bowl and stir in the corn.

Use about 1/2 cup of the batter per waffle and bake according to the manufacturer's directions.

Chef's Note

Leftover waffles can be frozen for up to 2 weeks; just reheat them in the toaster oven.

Three-Berry Compote recipe on page 359

PREPARATION TIME
10 minutes

BAKING TIME
30 minutes

Blueberry Clafouti

serves 6

Clafouti is a French dessert often made with cherries. But you may substitute other fruit, such as the blueberries used here, pears, other berries or fresh figs.

2½	cups blueberries
1	cup fat-free egg substitute
⅔	cup skim milk
¼	cup honey
¼	cup whole-wheat flour
¼	cup all-purpose flour
1	tablespoon canola oil
½	teaspoon vanilla

Preheat the oven to 400°.

Coat a 9" pie plate with no-stick spray. Add the blueberries.

In a blender, process the egg substitute, milk, honey, whole-wheat flour, all-purpose flour, oil and vanilla until smooth. Pour over the blueberries.

Bake for 25 to 30 minutes, or until puffed and golden.

Cranberry Fruitcake

serves 10

This moist cake takes only a few minutes to ready for the oven. As with many other desserts in this chapter, you may vary the fruit. Try substituting pears for the apples and blueberries for the cranberries.

PREPARATION TIME
15 minutes

BAKING TIME
25 minutes

$^2/_3$	cup whole-wheat flour
$^2/_3$	cup all-purpose flour
$^1/_2$	cup rolled oats
$1^1/_2$	teaspoons baking soda
1	teaspoon ground ginger
$^1/_2$	cup fat-free egg substitute
$^1/_2$	cup honey
$^1/_3$	cup orange juice
$^1/_4$	cup canola oil
1	teaspoon vanilla
1	cup cranberries
$^3/_4$	cup shredded apples

Preheat the oven to 350°. Coat a 13" × 9" baking dish with no-stick spray.

In a large bowl, whisk together the whole-wheat flour, all-purpose flour, oats, baking soda and ginger.

In a medium bowl, whisk together the egg substitute, honey, orange juice, oil and vanilla. Pour over the flour mixture and stir until just incorporated; do not overmix. Stir in the cranberries and apples.

Spread the batter evenly in the baking dish. Bake for 20 to 25 minutes, or until a toothpick inserted in the center comes out clean. Cool on a wire rack.

PREPARATION TIME
10 minutes

BAKING TIME
50 minutes

Gingerbread

serves 12

Serve this old-fashioned cake plain or with fat-free whipped topping.

1¼	cups all-purpose flour
1	cup whole-wheat flour
1½	teaspoons ground ginger
1	teaspoon baking soda
1	teaspoon ground cinnamon
¼	teaspoon ground allspice
1	cup hot water
½	cup molasses
½	cup honey
6	tablespoons canola oil
¼	cup fat-free egg substitute

Preheat the oven to 325°. Coat an 8" × 8" baking dish with no-stick spray.

In a large bowl, whisk together the all-purpose flour, whole-wheat flour, ginger, baking soda, cinnamon and allspice.

In a medium bowl, whisk together the water, molasses, honey, oil and egg substitute. Pour over the flour mixture and beat until smooth.

Pour the batter into the baking dish. Bake for 50 minutes, or until a toothpick inserted in the center comes out clean. Cool on a wire rack.

Dried Cherry Whole-Wheat Loaf

makes 1 loaf (18 slices)

Sour Montmorency is the most popular cherry for drying. Drying deepens its bright red color and concentrates the tart flavor. Dried cherries add texture and lovely color to this quick-to-fix filled bread.

Flour

1 loaf frozen whole-wheat dough, defrosted according to the manufacturer's directions

¼ cup all-fruit cherry spread

½ cup dried cherries

2 teaspoons almond extract

2 tablespoons skim milk

PREPARATION TIME
5 minutes
plus 30 minutes
rising time

BAKING TIME
35 minutes

Lightly flour the work surface. Roll the dough into an 11" × 7" rectangle. Place the cherry spread over the surface of the dough, stopping 1" from all the edges.

In a small bowl, combine the dried cherries with the almond extract. Sprinkle over the fruit spread. Starting at one 7" side, roll the dough into a cylinder. Firmly press the edges of the loaf together. (Water pressed on the seam helps keep the seal.)

Coat a 9" × 5" loaf pan with no-stick spray. Place the loaf in the prepared pan, seam side down. Brush with the milk. Cover with plastic wrap and let rise for 30 minutes. Bake at 375° for 30 to 35 minutes, or until the loaf is golden brown and a toothpick inserted in the center comes out clean.

Chef's Note

For other variations of this bread, substitute any dried fruit and its matching all-fruit spread for the dried cherries and cherry spread.

For a round loaf, shape the bread into a 12"- to 14"-long cylinder. Bake it in a tube or angel food cake pan coated with no-stick spray.

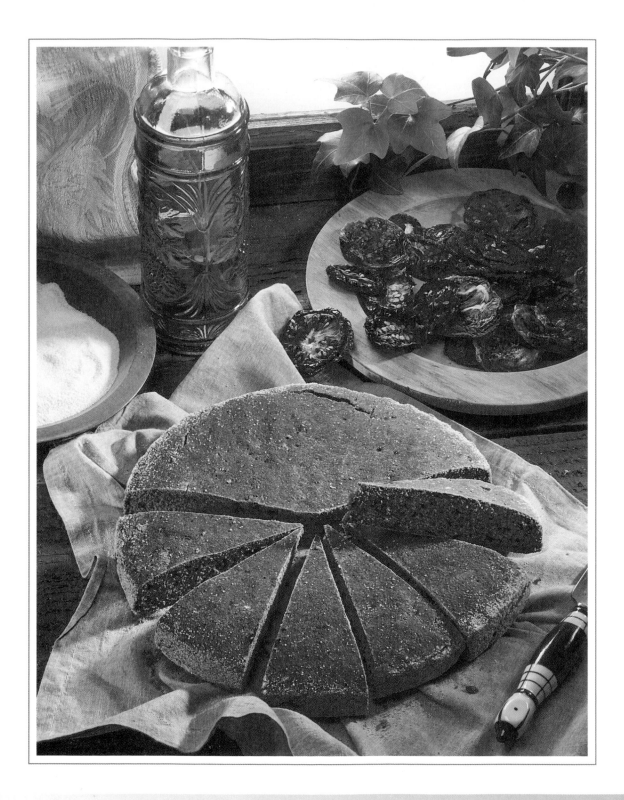

Sun-Dried Tomato Semolina Bread

makes 1 loaf (10 wedges)

Semolina is a coarsely ground flour made from durum wheat. It gives this bread, flecked with bits of sun-dried tomatoes, a chewy, hearty texture.

8	sun-dried tomato halves
1	cup boiling water
1	cup semolina flour
1/2	cup cornmeal
2	teaspoons dried oregano
2	teaspoons baking powder
1/2	teaspoon baking soda
1/2–1	cup all-purpose flour
1	cup tomato juice
2	tablespoons olive oil

Preheat the oven to 400°. Coat a 9" cake pan with no-stick spray.

In a small bowl, combine the tomatoes and water. Let stand for 5 minutes. Drain and coarsely chop.

In a food processor, combine the semolina flour, cornmeal, oregano, baking powder, baking soda and 1/2 cup of the all-purpose flour. Mix using on/off turns.

Add the tomato juice, oil and tomatoes. Mix using on/off turns and adding enough of the remaining all-purpose flour to form a soft dough.

With lightly floured hands, press the dough into the pan. Bake for 30 to 35 minutes, or until a toothpick inserted in the center comes out clean.

PER WEDGE

148 calories

3.3 g. fat
(16% of calories)

1.8 g. dietary fiber

0 mg. cholesterol

202 mg. sodium

PREPARATION TIME
10 minutes

BAKING TIME
35 minutes

PREPARATION TIME
15 minutes

BAKING TIME
25 minutes

Focaccia

makes 1 loaf (8 wedges)

Focaccia is the flat bread of Italy. Before being baked, the dough is often deeply poked with a finger to hold herbs, olive oil and any number of other ingredients. Focaccia bread is generally served warm or at room temperature but never sizzling hot like pizza.

1	cup warm water (120°)
1	package quick-rise yeast
1	teaspoon honey
2½–3	cups all-purpose flour
1	tablespoon chopped fresh rosemary
1	tablespoon chopped fresh sage
1½	teaspoons salt
3	tablespoons olive oil

Preheat the oven to 400°. Coat a large baking sheet with no-stick spray.

In a large bowl, whisk together the water, yeast and honey. Whisk in 1 cup of the flour and beat until smooth. Let stand for 5 minutes.

Beat in the rosemary, sage, salt, 2 tablespoons of the oil and 1 cup of the remaining flour. Beat for 3 minutes, or until smooth. Beat in enough of the remaining flour to form a soft, sticky dough.

Turn the dough out onto a lightly floured surface and knead for 3 minutes.

Transfer to the baking sheet and shape into a 9" round about 1" thick. Brush with the remaining 1 tablespoon oil.

Bake for 20 to 25 minutes, or until golden brown.

American Harvest Loaf

makes 1 loaf (12 wedges)

You'll be glad you spent the time baking this wonderfully flavorful and versatile bread. It freezes well and makes great toast. Cut slices into cubes and dry them for crunchy croutons to sprinkle on soups or salads.

PER WEDGE

58 calories

0.7 g. fat
(11% of calories)

0.9 g. dietary fiber

0 mg. cholesterol

15 mg. sodium

½	cup cracked wheat
1	cup boiling water
1	cup whole-wheat flour
¼	cup oat bran
¼	cup sunflower seeds
1	package quick-rise yeast
¼	teaspoon salt
2	cups all-purpose flour
¾	cup warm water (120°)
2	tablespoons honey

PREPARATION TIME
15 minutes
plus 40 minutes
rising time

BAKING TIME
35 minutes

Photo on page 83

In a small bowl, mix the cracked wheat and boiling water. Let stand for 10 minutes.

In a large bowl, whisk together the whole-wheat flour, oat bran, sunflower seeds, yeast, salt and 1 cup of the all-purpose flour.

In a cup, mix the warm water and honey. Pour over the flour mixture. Add the undrained cracked wheat. Beat until the dough forms a rough-looking mass.

Turn the dough out onto a lightly floured surface and knead in enough of the remaining all-purpose flour to form a soft dough. Knead for 5 minutes.

Coat a large bowl with no-stick spray. Place the dough in the bowl. Cover with plastic wrap and allow to rise for 10 minutes. Press the dough to eliminate any air bubbles. Shape into a 12" round.

Coat a large baking sheet with no-stick spray. Place the loaf on the sheet. Mist the top with no-stick spray. Cover with plastic wrap. Let rise for 30 minutes, or until doubled in size.

Bake at 350° for 35 minutes, or until a toothpick inserted in the center comes out clean.

Sweet Temptations

DELECTABLE DESSERTS
THAT ARE GOOD FOR YOU

In this chapter, we've gathered a host of luscious sweets. Some of the desserts were inspired by and borrowed from the diverse cultures that make up this country. There are biscotti and cannoli from Italy, strudel from Germany, fruity clafouti from France and more. But we've also created lots of all-American sweet traditions—like cherry pie, chocolate cake, carrot cake, cheesecake and rice pudding. Now if you're thinking that these desserts are off your eating list because they're high in fat, think again! We've reduced the fat in each and every one so you can enjoy them often.

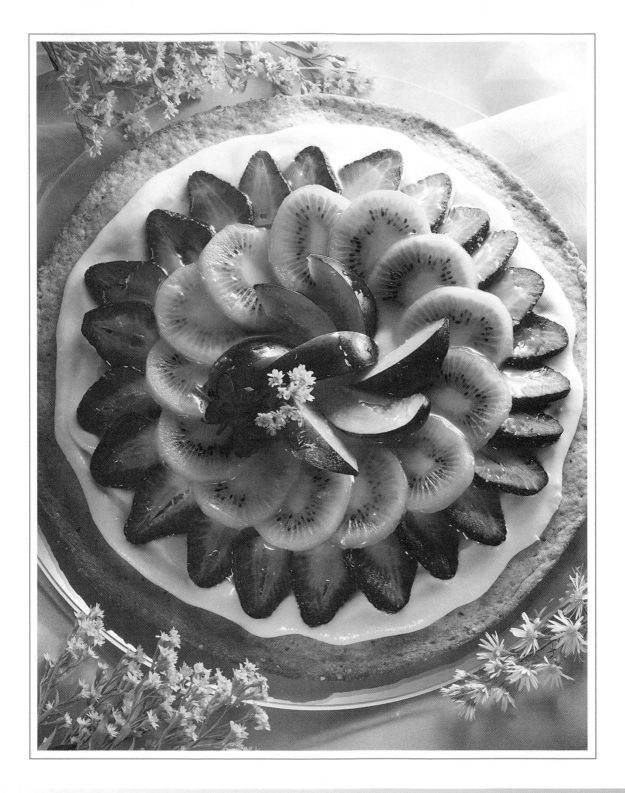

Summertime Fruit Pizza

serves 8

What a novel way to turn a classic main course into dessert! Feel free to improvise with whatever fruit you have on hand.

1	cup all-purpose flour
3	tablespoons sugar
2	tablespoons finely chopped almonds
1/4	cup low-fat buttermilk
2	tablespoons canola oil
8	ounces reduced-fat cream cheese, softened
1/2	cup confectioners' sugar
1	teaspoon grated orange rind
3	kiwifruit, sliced
1	cup sliced strawberries
1	nectarine, sliced
1/2	cup apple jelly, melted

PREPARATION TIME
10 minutes
plus 30 minutes
chilling time

BAKING TIME
12 minutes

In a large bowl, whisk together the flour, sugar, and almonds. Stir in the buttermilk and oil. Form into a ball, flatten, wrap in plastic wrap and refrigerate for at least 30 minutes.

Preheat the oven to 375°. Coat a pizza pan with no-stick spray.

Unwrap the dough and place it between pieces of wax paper. Gently roll into a circle about 1/8" thick. Remove the top piece of wax paper. Invert the dough onto the pan. Remove the remaining piece of wax paper.

Bake for 12 minutes, or until lightly browned. Cool on a wire rack.

In a medium bowl, beat together the cream cheese, confectioners' sugar and orange rind. Spread over the crust. Arrange the kiwifruit, strawberries and nectarines on top. Brush with the jelly.

PREPARATION TIME
20 minutes

BAKING TIME
50 minutes

Carrot Cake

serves 16

Each bite of this cake is rich, moist and spicy.

1¾	cups all-purpose flour
1	cup whole-wheat flour
2	teaspoons baking powder
2	teaspoons baking soda
2	teaspoons ground cinnamon
1	teaspoon ground nutmeg
¾	teaspoon ground allspice
¼	teaspoon salt
2	eggs
4	egg whites
1	cup packed brown sugar
1	cup fat-free plain yogurt
¼	cup canola oil
2	cups grated carrots
1	cup drained canned crushed pineapple
⅔	cup currants
8	ounces reduced-fat cream cheese, softened
1	box (16 ounces) confectioners' sugar
2	teaspoons vanilla

Preheat the oven to 325°. Coat a 13" × 9" baking dish with no-stick spray.

In a medium bowl, whisk together the all-purpose flour, whole-wheat flour, baking powder, baking soda, cinnamon, nutmeg, allspice and salt. In a large bowl, beat the eggs and egg whites with an electric mixer on medium speed until foamy. Add the brown sugar. Beat for 3 minutes. Add the yogurt and oil. Beat until creamy. On low speed, beat in the flour mixture. Gently stir in the carrots, pineapple and currants. Spread in the baking dish.

Bake for 40 to 50 minutes, or until a toothpick inserted in the center comes out clean. Cool on a wire rack.

In a large bowl, beat the cream cheese, confectioners' sugar and vanilla until smooth. Spread over the cooled cake.

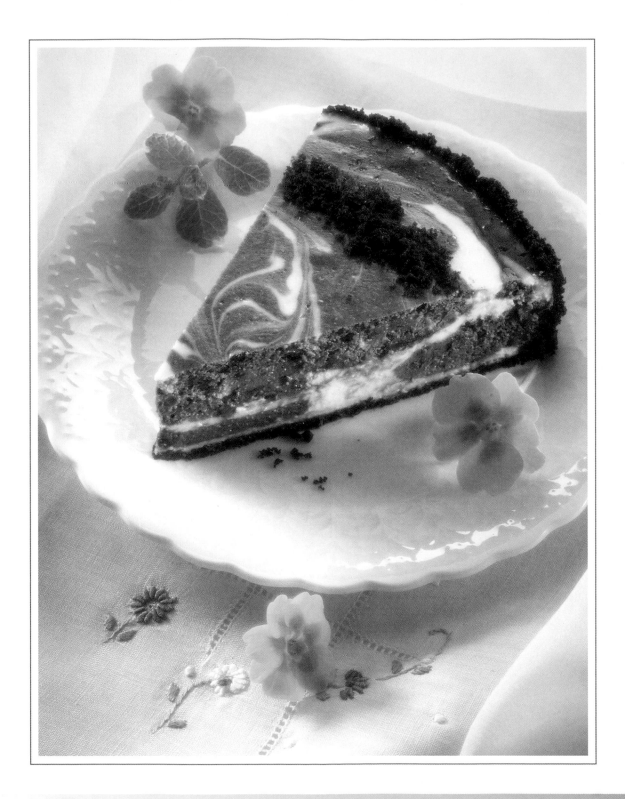

Chocolate-Orange Swirl Cheesecake

serves 12

Say yes to cheesecake when it's this low in fat—and super delicious in the bargain!

PER SERVING
293 calories

7.6 g. fat
(30% of calories)

1.8 g. dietary fiber

38 mg. cholesterol

323 mg. sodium

1½	cups chocolate cookie crumbs
8	ounces reduced-fat cream cheese, softened
1	cup low-fat ricotta cheese
2	eggs
3	tablespoons cornstarch
1	tablespoon grated orange rind
¾	cup plus 2 tablespoons sugar
¼	cup unsweetened cocoa powder

PREPARATION TIME
10 minutes

BAKING TIME
30 minutes

Preheat the oven to 400°.

Coat a 9" pie plate with no-stick spray. Press the cookie crumbs evenly over the bottom and up the sides.

In a large bowl, beat together the cream cheese and ricotta until smooth. Stir in the eggs, cornstarch, orange rind and ¾ cup of the sugar.

Pour half of the mixture into another bowl. Stir in the cocoa powder and the remaining 2 tablespoons sugar. Pour into the pie plate.

Spoon the remaining cheese mixture over the top and swirl with a knife to achieve a marbleized effect.

Bake for 30 minutes, or until a knife inserted in the center comes out clean.

Chef's Note
You may substitute graham cracker crumbs for the chocolate cookie crumbs.

PREPARATION TIME
10 minutes

BAKING TIME
30 minutes

New York Cheesecake

serves 12

Reduced-fat cream cheese and a skinny cookie crust are the secrets to this light treat. For a lovely presentation, garnish with fresh fruit.

1/3	cup amaretti cookie crumbs
8	ounces reduced-fat cream cheese, softened
1	cup reduced-fat ricotta cheese
1/4	cup honey
3	tablespoons cornstarch
1	tablespoon grated orange rind
2	eggs, separated

Preheat the oven to 400°.

Coat a 9" pie plate with no-stick spray. Press the cookie crumbs evenly over the bottom and up the sides.

In a large bowl, beat together the cream cheese and ricotta until smooth. Stir in the honey, cornstarch, orange rind and egg yolks.

In a medium bowl, whip the egg whites with clean beaters until soft peaks form. Fold into the cream cheese mixture. Pour into the pie plate.

Bake for 30 minutes, or until a knife inserted in the center comes out clean.

Chef's Note

You may substitute graham cracker crumbs for the amaretti crumbs.

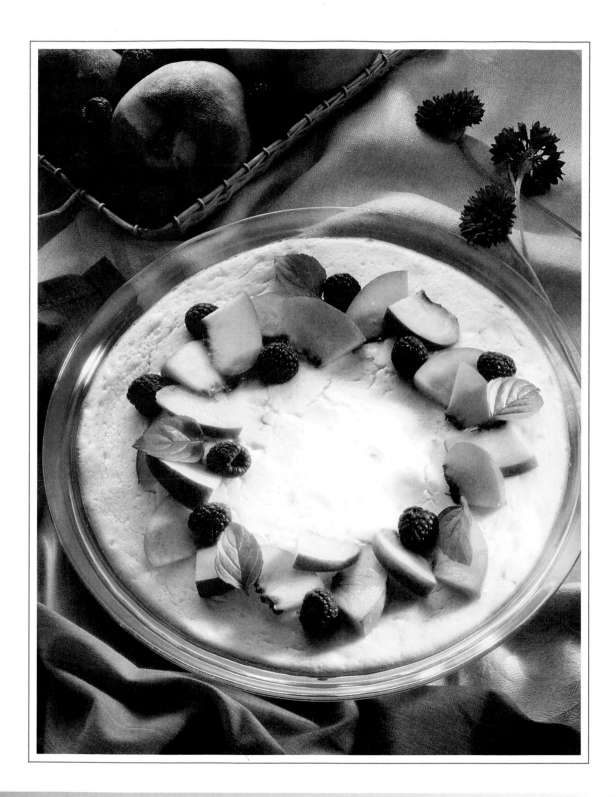

PREPARATION TIME
10 minutes

BAKING TIME
32 minutes

Citrus Ricotta Cannoli

makes 20

True Italian cannoli are light and zesty with a creamy mascarpone filling. In this recipe, the cannoli shells are baked (not fried), and whipped fat-free ricotta replaces the fat-laden mascarpone cheese. These are wonderful on a dessert platter for a buffet.

Cannoli Shells

1/3	cup sugar
2	tablespoons butter or margarine, melted
2	egg whites
1/2	teaspoon almond extract
1/2	teaspoon vanilla
1/3	cup all-purpose flour

Citrus Ricotta Filling

1	container (15 ounces) fat-free ricotta cheese
1/4	cup sugar
1	tablespoon grated orange rind
2	teaspoons grated lemon rind
1	teaspoon grated lime rind
1	teaspoon vanilla
1	ounce bittersweet chocolate, finely chopped

TO MAKE THE CANNOLI SHELLS
Preheat the oven to 375°. Coat 2 baking sheets with no-stick spray.

In a large bowl, stir together the sugar and butter or margarine. Stir in the egg whites, almond extract and vanilla. Stir in the flour.

Place 3 mounds of batter (1 tablespoon each) on each baking sheet; spread each mound into a very thin 4" circle.

Bake for 6 to 8 minutes, or until set. Using a spatula, gently lift the cannoli off the sheets and wrap around thick dowels or cannoli molds. Cool, then slide off the molds. Repeat until all the batter is used.

TO MAKE THE CITRUS RICOTTA FILLING

In a medium bowl, combine the ricotta, sugar, orange rind, lemon rind, lime rind and vanilla. Beat with an electric mixer on medium speed until smooth. Stir in the chocolate.

Spoon the filling into the cannoli shells.

Chef's Note

The shells and filling may be made several days in advance. Store the shells in an airtight container; keep the filling in a covered container in the refrigerator. Assemble just before serving.

Three-Berry Compote

serves 4

Most any fresh berries would work in this recipe. Serve as is or use as a topping for pancakes, waffles, frozen yogurt or angel food cake.

1	cup blueberries
1	cup raspberries
1	cup boysenberries or blackberries
1/4	cup maple syrup
1/4	teaspoon ground nutmeg
1/2	teaspoon grated orange rind

In a medium bowl, mix the blueberries, raspberries, boysenberries or blackberries, maple syrup, nutmeg and orange rind. Let marinate at room temperature for 30 minutes.

Chef's Note

If fresh berries are unavailable, use thawed frozen ones.

PER SERVING

101 calories

0.4 g. fat
(4% of calories)

3.7 g. dietary fiber

0 mg. cholesterol

5 mg. sodium

PREPARATION TIME
5 minutes
plus 30 minutes
marinating time

Photo on page 339

Quick Chocolate Cake

serves 12

This rich-tasting snack cake has old-fashioned chocolate flavor, yet it's very light, thanks to the buttermilk. Extra pieces make great lunchbox treats.

PER SERVING

235 calories

4.9 g. fat
(18% of calories)

0.7 g. dietary fiber

27 mg. cholesterol

152 mg. sodium

1 cup all-purpose flour

1/2 cup unsweetened cocoa powder

1 teaspoon ground cinnamon

1/2 teaspoon ground nutmeg

1/2 teaspoon baking powder

1/2 teaspoon baking soda

1 cup packed brown sugar

1/2 cup applesauce

2 tablespoons canola oil

1 tablespoon vanilla

1 egg

1/2 cup low-fat buttermilk

2 egg whites

Confectioner's sugar

PREPARATION TIME
15 minutes

BAKING TIME
30 minutes

Preheat the oven to 350°. Coat an 8" × 8" baking dish with no-stick spray.

In medium bowl, whisk together the flour, cocoa powder, cinnamon, nutmeg, baking powder and baking soda.

In a large bowl, whisk together the brown sugar, applesauce, oil, vanilla and egg. Alternately beat in the flour mixture and the buttermilk, beginning and ending with the flour mixture.

In a small bowl, whip the egg whites with clean beaters until soft peaks form. Fold into the batter. Pour into the baking dish.

Bake for 25 to 30 minutes, or until a toothpick inserted in the center comes out clean. Cool on a wire rack. Dust with confectioner's sugar before slicing.

PREPARATION TIME
25 minutes

BAKING TIME
40 minutes

Sweetheart Cherry Pie

serves 4

Who doesn't love cherry pie! This pretty, low-fat version is decorated with pastry hearts.

Cherry Filling

4	cups pitted sour cherries
1/2	cup maple syrup
3	tablespoons quick-cooking tapioca
1	teaspoon ground cinnamon

Pie Crust

1	cup cake flour
1/4	cup butter or margarine, cut into small pieces
1	egg white

TO MAKE THE CHERRY FILLING
In a 2-quart saucepan, mix the cherries, maple syrup, tapioca and cinnamon. Let stand for 5 minutes. Cook over medium heat for 10 minutes, stirring occasionally.

TO MAKE THE PIE CRUST
Preheat the oven to 400°.

Place the flour in a medium bowl. Using 2 knives, cut in the butter or margarine until the mixture resembles coarse meal. Stir in the egg white. Transfer to a lightly floured surface and knead for 30 seconds, or until smooth.

Reserve 1/4 cup of the dough. Place the remaining dough between sheets of wax paper and roll into a 9" circle. Remove the top piece of wax paper. Invert the dough onto an 8" pie plate. Remove the remaining piece of wax paper and fit the dough into the pie plate. Fold under the excess pastry and crimp the edges. Prick the bottom of the dough and bake for 10 minutes.

Roll the reserved dough between sheets of wax paper to 1/8" thickness. Using a cookie cutter, cut out hearts or other decorative shapes.

Pour the cherry filling into the pie crust and arrange the cutouts on top. Reduce the oven temperature to 350°. Bake for 30 minutes.

Chef's Note
You may use frozen sour cherries that have been thawed instead of fresh cherries.

Sweet Temptations

Rustic Plum-Walnut Tart

serves 6

This free-form tart makes delicious use of beautiful late-summer plums. The crust absorbs the luscious plum juices, yet stays crisp and light.

PER SERVING
244 calories
6.2 g. fat (22% of calories)
1.7 g. dietary fiber
0 mg. cholesterol
123 mg. sodium

PREPARATION TIME
20 minutes

BAKING TIME
45 minutes

Crust

1	cup all-purpose flour
1	tablespoon sugar
1/4	teaspoon salt
1/4	teaspoon ground cinnamon
2	tablespoons canola oil
3–4	tablespoons ice water

Plum Filling

4	tablespoons low-fat granola
2	tablespoons all-purpose flour
2	tablespoons chopped toasted walnuts
1/3	cup plus 1 teaspoon sugar
6	plums, quartered
1	tablespoon skim milk
2	tablespoons red currant jelly

TO MAKE THE CRUST
In a medium bowl, whisk together the flour, sugar, salt and cinnamon. Using a fork, slowly stir in the oil until the mixture is crumbly. Stir in enough of the ice water to form a dough that holds together. (It will be a little wetter than traditional pastry dough.)

Place the dough between sheets of wax paper and roll into a 12" circle. Remove the top piece of wax paper. Invert the dough onto a baking sheet. Remove the remaining piece of wax paper.

TO MAKE THE PLUM FILLING
Preheat the oven to 400°.

In a food processor, process the granola, flour, walnuts and 1/3 cup of the sugar until finely ground. Spread over the dough, leaving about a 2" border.

(continued)

Decoratively arrange the plums on top of the granola mixture. Fold the dough border over the plums. Brush the milk over the dough and sprinkle with the remaining 1 teaspoon sugar.

Bake for 30 to 40 minutes, or until the crust is golden and the plums are tender. With a long metal spatula, loosen the pastry bottom. Slide the tart onto a platter and let cool.

Melt the jelly in a 1-quart saucepan over low heat. Brush over the plums.

Chef's Note

Use seasonal fruit when preparing this tart. Peaches work well in the summer. Apples or pears are delicious in fall and winter.

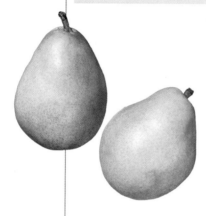

Pear and Raisin Strudel

serves 8

This easy-to-assemble strudel is made with phyllo dough, which is available in the freezer section of most supermarkets. Traditional phyllo recipes use lots of butter to make the pastry layers crisp. But this strudel gets the same results with just a fraction of the fat by using a light coat of no-stick spray between the layers.

PER SERVING

147 calories

1.8 g. fat
(11% of calories)

1.6 g. dietary fiber

0 mg. cholesterol

3 mg. sodium

PREPARATION TIME
15 minutes

BAKING TIME
35 minutes

2½	cups thinly sliced pears
½	cup raisins
⅓	cup maple syrup
1	tablespoon lemon juice
¼	teaspoon ground cinnamon
¼	teaspoon ground nutmeg
8	sheets phyllo dough

Preheat the oven to 350°. Coat a large baking sheet with no-stick spray.

In a large bowl, mix the pears, raisins, maple syrup, lemon juice, cinnamon and nutmeg.

Unroll the phyllo and cover with a barely damp towel to keep the sheets from drying out.

Peel off 1 phyllo sheet and place it on a work surface; re-cover the remainder. Lightly coat the top of the sheet with no-stick spray. Cover with a second sheet and brush very lightly with water. Repeat the process, coating alternate sheets with either spray or water, until all sheets have been used.

Spoon the pear mixture onto the dough; position it on the bottom half of the rectangle and leave a 1" border on the sides and bottom. Fold in the sides and roll the sheets to enclose the pear mixture.

Transfer the roll, seam side down, to the baking sheet. Lightly brush the top with water. Bake for 30 to 35 minutes, or until golden.

PREPARATION TIME
10 minutes

BAKING TIME
20 minutes

Oven-Puffed Pancake

serves 4

The Dutch call them pannekoeken. You'll just call them fabulous. For the most dramatic "puff," cook the pancake in a wide pan.

³⁄₄	cup fat-free egg substitute
¹⁄₂	cup skim milk
2	tablespoons canola oil
2	teaspoons vanilla
1	teaspoon ground nutmeg
¹⁄₂	cup all-purpose flour
2	tablespoons packed brown sugar
2	tablespoons lemon juice

Preheat the oven to 450°. Coat a large ovenproof frying pan or cast-iron skillet with no-stick spray.

In a medium bowl, whisk together the egg substitute, milk, oil, vanilla and nutmeg. Slowly whisk in the flour to form a smooth batter. Pour into the pan.

Cook over medium heat for 2 minutes to set the batter. Bake for 15 minutes. Reduce the oven temperature to 350° and bake for 5 minutes, or until puffed and golden brown.

Sprinkle with the brown sugar and lemon juice. Serve immediately.

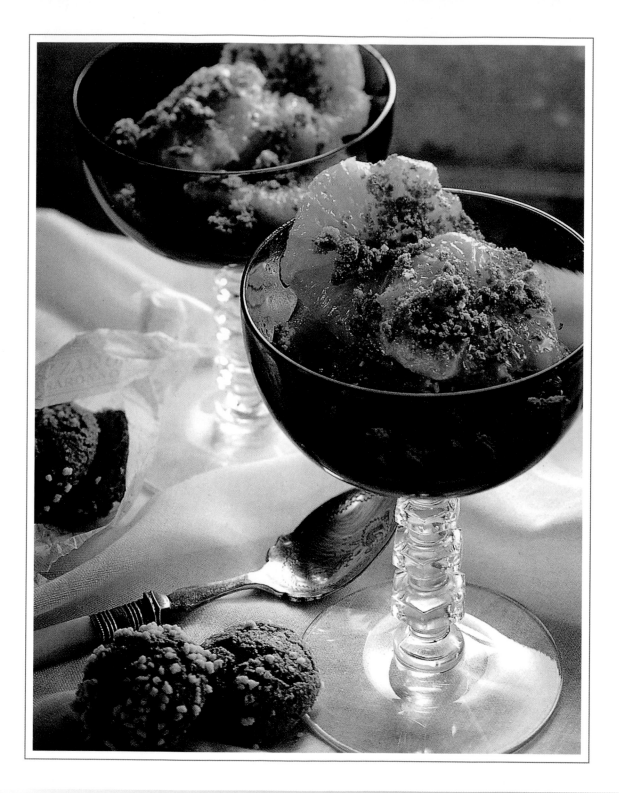

Sautéed Oranges with Amaretti Cookies

serves 4

PER SERVING
199 calories
4.4 g. fat (21% of calories)
4.3 g. dietary fiber
3 mg. cholesterol
38 mg. sodium

Amaretti cookies are widely available in supermarkets and Italian specialty stores. To crush them, place in a heavy plastic bag and use a rolling pin.

4	large navel oranges, peeled and sliced crosswise
1	teaspoon butter or margarine
2	tablespoons packed brown sugar
1	teaspoon frozen orange juice concentrate, thawed
²/₃	cup crushed amaretti cookies

In a large no-stick frying pan over medium-high heat, cook the oranges, butter or margarine, brown sugar and orange juice concentrate for 3 minutes, or until the oranges soften slightly. Sprinkle with the cookie crumbs.

PREPARATION TIME
10 minutes

COOKING TIME
3 minutes

PREPARATION TIME
5 minutes

COOKING TIME
3 minutes

Grilled Summer Fruit with Berry Sauce

serves 4

Grilling brings out the sweet flavors of fruit. And the bright raspberry sauce gives it a crowning touch of color and flavor.

1	cup raspberries
1	tablespoon packed brown sugar
1½	teaspoons lemon juice
2	apricots, halved
2	plums, halved
1	peach, halved
1	teaspoon canola oil
2	teaspoons honey

In a blender or food processor, process the raspberries, brown sugar and lemon juice until smooth. If desired, strain out the seeds.

Brush the cut sides of the apricot, plum and peach halves with the oil. Grill the fruit, oiled side down, for 2 to 3 minutes, or until lightly browned. Remove from the grill and drizzle with the honey. Serve topped with the raspberry sauce.

PREPARATION TIME
10 minutes

BAKING TIME
10 minutes

Broiled Pineapple
with Papaya Puree

serves 4

Any tropical fruit broils beautifully and can be substituted for the pineapple in this fast dessert. Mango can replace the papaya in the puree.

1	can (8 ounces) pineapple rings packed in juice, drained
3	tablespoons lime juice
2	cups chopped papaya
2	tablespoons maple syrup
	Pinch of ground nutmeg
½	cup fat-free plain yogurt

Place the pineapple rings on a broiler pan and drizzle with 2 tablespoons of the lime juice. Broil 4" from the heat for 2 to 5 minutes, or until light brown. Turn and broil for 2 to 5 minutes.

In a blender or food processor, process the papaya, maple syrup, nutmeg and the remaining 1 tablespoon lime juice until smooth. Serve over the pineapple. Top with dollops of the yogurt.

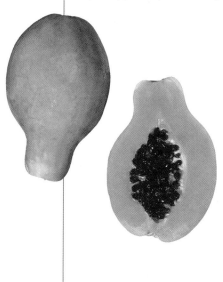

Mandarin Rice Pudding

serves 6

Here's an easy rice pudding that gets Asian flair from mandarin oranges and crystallized ginger. For an even more intriguing flavor, start with an aromatic rice, such as basmati. This pudding is good warm or chilled.

PER SERVING

217 calories

3.3 g. fat
(14% of calories)

0.6 g. dietary fiber

3 mg. cholesterol

88 mg. sodium

PREPARATION TIME
5 minutes

COOKING TIME
35 minutes

1	cup rice
2	teaspoons canola oil
2	cups water
1/4	teaspoon ground cinnamon
1	can (15 ounces) evaporated skim milk
1	cup drained and chopped mandarin oranges
2	tablespoons minced crystallized ginger
2	tablespoons toasted almonds

In a 3-quart saucepan over medium heat, stir the rice and oil for 3 minutes, or until glossy. Stir in the water and cinnamon. Bring to a boil. Cover, reduce the heat to medium-low and simmer for 20 minutes, or until all the liquid has been absorbed.

Stir in the milk. Cook, stirring often, for 10 minutes. Stir in the oranges, ginger and almonds.

Strawberries
in Raspberry Puree

serves 4

Plump, juicy strawberries are drenched in a brilliant raspberry sauce. Serve this beautiful combination in long-stemmed goblets, garnished with mint leaves.

2	cups raspberries
2	tablespoons sugar
1/4	teaspoon almond extract
1	pint strawberries

In a food processor, process the raspberries, sugar and almond extract until smooth. If desired, strain out the seeds. Pour over the strawberries and allow to marinate for 15 minutes.

Chef's Note

You may use fresh or frozen raspberries in the puree.
If you use frozen berries, thaw them before processing.

Chocolate-Walnut Biscotti recipe on page 382

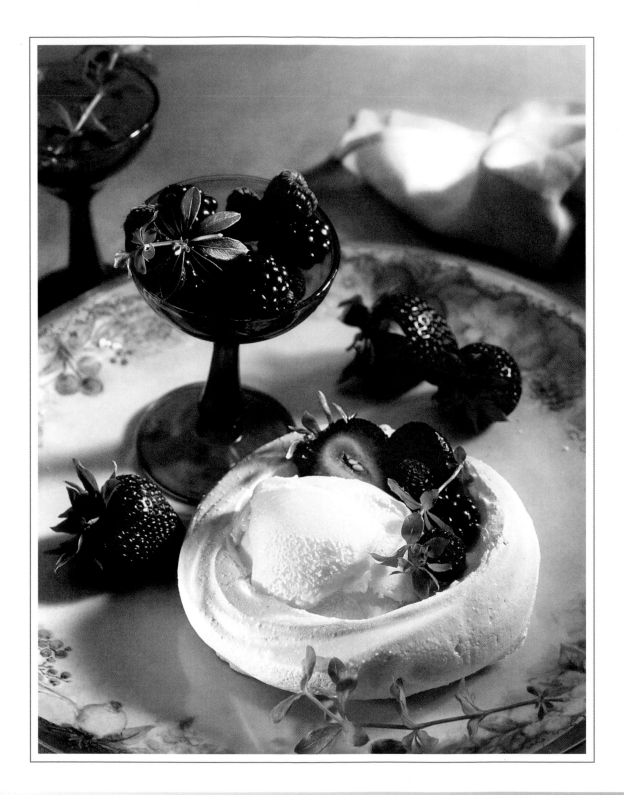

Sweet Temptations

Meringues with Lemon Sorbet and Berries

serves 4

PER SERVING

268 calories

2.8 g. fat
(9% of calories)

1.9 g. dietary fiber

0 mg. cholesterol

143 mg. sodium

These meringue shells are crisp and dry, a heavenly contrast to the tart sorbet and sweet berries. Use a mixture of whatever berries are in season, such as blackberries, raspberries, blueberries or strawberries.

Meringue Shells

3	egg whites
1/4	teaspoon cream of tartar
1/8	teaspoon salt
3/4	cup sugar
1/2	teaspoon vanilla
1/2	teaspoon lemon juice

Filling

2	cups berries
1	tablespoon sugar
2	cups lemon sorbet

PREPARATION TIME
10 minutes

BAKING TIME
1 hour
plus 1 hour
standing time

TO MAKE THE MERINGUE SHELLS
Preheat the oven to 225°. Cover a large baking sheet with parchment paper.

In a large bowl, combine the egg whites, cream of tartar and salt. Beat with an electric mixer on medium speed until soft peaks form. Gradually beat in the sugar, 1 tablespoon at a time, until the meringue is stiff and shiny. Beat in the vanilla and lemon juice.

Drop 4 large spoonfuls of meringue, evenly spaced, on the baking sheet. With the back of a spoon, form the meringue into little nests.

Bake for 1 hour. Turn the oven off and let the meringues stand with the door closed for 1 hour. Cool on a wire rack.

TO MAKE THE FILLING
In a small bowl, toss the berries with the sugar. Divide the sorbet among the meringue shells and top with the berries.

Chef's Note
Meringues may be made ahead and stored in an airtight container for up to 2 weeks.

Mango Sorbet

serves 4

PREPARATION TIME
5 minutes
plus freezing time

True sorbet contains no milk, making it virtually fat-free. Mangoes give this icy-smooth dessert its brilliant orange color and sweet-tangy flavor.

    1   can (15 ounces) mangoes, drained and pureed
    1/2 cup carbonated water
    1/3 cup honey
    1   tablespoon lime juice

In a medium bowl, mix the mango puree, water, honey and lime juice. Transfer to an ice cream maker and freeze according to the manufacturer's directions.

PREPARATION TIME
10 minutes

BAKING TIME
25 minutes

Photo on page 377

Chocolate-Walnut Biscotti

makes 30

Dark and rich-tasting, these biscotti keep well in an air-tight container or in the freezer. They are especially good dunked in espresso.

1	cup all-purpose flour
1/2	cup sugar
1/4	cup unsweetened cocoa powder
1/2	teaspoon baking powder
1/4	teaspoon baking soda
1/4	teaspoon salt
1	egg
1	egg white
1 1/2	teaspoons vanilla
2	ounces bittersweet chocolate, chopped
1/4	cup chopped toasted walnuts

Preheat the oven to 350°. Coat an 11" × 7" baking dish with no-stick spray.

In a large bowl, whisk together the flour, sugar, cocoa powder, baking powder, baking soda and salt.

In a medium bowl, whisk together the egg, egg white and vanilla. Pour over the flour mixture and stir well. Stir in the chocolate and walnuts.

Press the dough into the baking dish. Bake for 25 minutes, or until firm. Transfer to a wire rack and cut into 30 fingers. Cool before serving.

Chef's Note

To toast nuts, spread them on a baking sheet and bake at 400° for 10 minutes, or until lightly browned and fragrant. Do not let them burn.

Mocha-Almond Biscotti

makes 30

Mild chocolate and light almond flavor come together nicely in this crunchy cookie. Great for dunking.

1¼	cups all-purpose flour
½	cup sugar
½	teaspoon baking powder
¼	teaspoon baking soda
¼	teaspoon salt
1	egg
1	egg white
1	teaspoon vanilla
½	teaspoon almond extract
1	tablespoon instant coffee powder
1	tablespoon warm water
1	ounce unsweetened chocolate, melted
⅓	cup slivered toasted almonds

Preheat the oven to 350°. Coat an 11" × 7" baking dish with no-stick spray.

In a large bowl, whisk together the flour, sugar, baking powder, baking soda and salt.

In a medium bowl, whisk together the egg, egg white, vanilla and almond extract. In a cup, dissolve the coffee in the water; stir into the bowl. Stir in the chocolate. Pour over the flour mixture and stir well. Stir in the almonds.

Press the dough into the baking dish. Bake for 25 minutes, or until firm. Transfer to a wire rack and cut into 30 fingers. Cool before serving.

PER BISCOTTI

73 calories

2.2 g. fat
(26% of calories)

0 g. dietary fiber

11 mg. cholesterol

52 mg. sodium

PREPARATION TIME
10 minutes

BAKING TIME
25 minutes

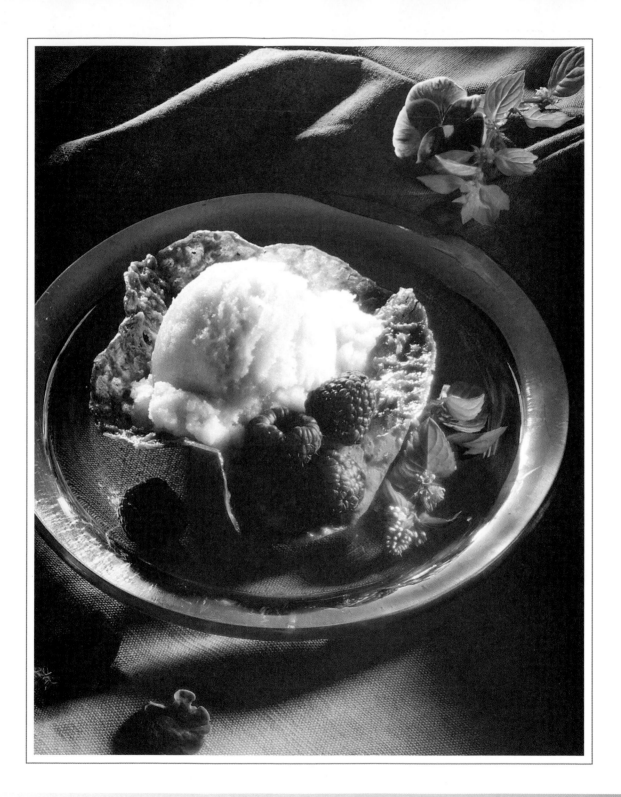

Sweet Temptations

Praline Cookie Cups

makes 8

Fill these thin, buttery, nutty cups with fresh berries or low-fat frozen yogurt.

PER CUP

93 calories

4.2 g. fat
(40% of calories)

0.3 g. dietary fiber

8 mg. cholesterol

6 mg. sodium

- ¼ cup all-purpose flour
- ¼ cup packed brown sugar
- 2 tablespoons butter or margarine, softened
- 2 tablespoons light corn syrup
- 2 tablespoons chopped toasted hazelnuts

PREPARATION TIME
5 minutes

BAKING TIME
7 minutes

Preheat the oven to 375°. Coat a large baking sheet with no-stick spray.

In a medium bowl, mix the flour, brown sugar, butter or margarine, corn syrup and hazelnuts. Divide the dough into 8 pieces and form into balls.

Place the balls 3" apart on the baking sheet and press lightly to flatten.

Bake for 5 to 7 minutes, or until lightly browned.

Cool on the baking sheet for 2 minutes. Loosen gently with a spatula and drape the warm cookies over the bottoms of custard cups. Let cool.

PREPARATION TIME
10 minutes

BAKING TIME
20 minutes

Baked Winter Fruit

serves 4

Baking fruit concentrates its natural sweetness and creates a moist, tender dessert. For a finishing touch, top the fruit with pureed frozen strawberries and fat-free vanilla frozen yogurt.

2	tart apples, cored, peeled and sliced into 4 rings each
2	pears, quartered
16	dried apricot halves
1	tablespoon currants
1	tablespoon red wine or apple juice
1	teaspoon maple syrup
½	teaspoon ground cinnamon

Preheat the oven to 400°. Tear off 4 large sheets of aluminum foil. Divide the apples, pears, apricots and currants evenly among the pieces. Drizzle with the wine or apple juice and maple syrup, then sprinkle with the cinnamon. Seal the packets tightly. Place on baking sheets.

Bake for 20 minutes, or until the fruit is tender.

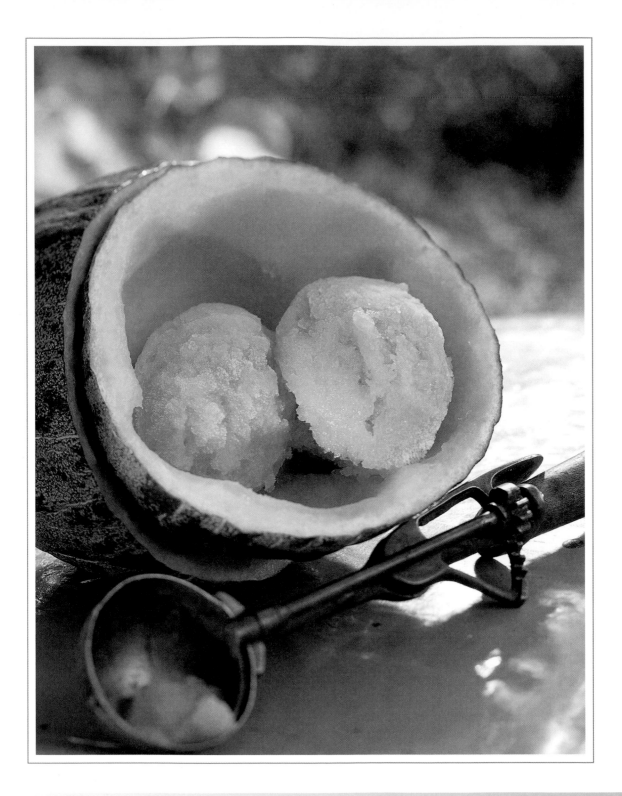

Sweet Temptations

Melon-Mango Sorbet

serves 4

PER SERVING

163 calories

0.4 g. fat
(2% of calories)

2.5 g. dietary fiber

0 mg. cholesterol

28 mg. sodium

Sorbet is one of the easiest—and most elegant—summer desserts. Serve in chilled margarita glasses, fresh fruit shells, or individual custard cups.

1	mango, cubed
2	cups frozen melon balls
$1/2$	cup sugar
$1/4$	cup lime juice

PREPARATION TIME
5 minutes
plus 40 minutes
freezing time

In a blender or food processor, process the mango, melon balls, sugar and lime juice until smooth. Pour into individual serving dishes, cover and freeze for 30 to 40 minutes, or until firm, stirring once to break up any ice crystals.

PREPARATION TIME
25 minutes
plus draining and
chilling time

BAKING TIME
10 minutes

Lemon Icebox Pie

serves 8

Good old-fashioned flavor prevails in this updated version of a traditional pie. The use of a graham cracker crust in place of a standard pie shell helps cut calories and fat. Although preparing the pie is easy, you'll want to allow plenty of time for the yogurt in the filling to drain and more time to let the finished pie chill.

1	cup fat-free plain yogurt
6	graham crackers
1	tablespoon canola oil
1/4	cup cornstarch
1/2	cup plus 1 tablespoon sugar
2	cups low-fat vanilla yogurt
1/2	cup fat-free egg substitute
1/2	cup lemon juice
1/2	teaspoon lemon extract
1/4	teaspoon almond extract
3	egg whites
1/2	teaspoon cream of tartar
1	teaspoon vanilla

Spoon the plain yogurt into a yogurt cheese funnel or a strainer lined with cheesecloth. Set over a tall glass. Cover, refrigerate and allow to drain for 8 hours, or until very thick.

In a food processor, grind the graham crackers into crumbs. Add the oil and process with on/off turns until just combined. Coat a 10" pie plate with no-stick spray. Press the crumbs into the pan to make a crust.

Preheat the oven to 325°.

In a 2-quart saucepan, whisk together the cornstarch and 1/2 cup of the sugar. Whisk in the vanilla yogurt and the drained plain yogurt. Cook over medium heat, stirring constantly, for 5 minutes, or until the mixture comes to a boil and thickens.

Remove from the heat. Slowly whisk in the egg substitute. Reduce the heat to low. Cook, stirring constantly, for 2 minutes. Remove from the heat and whisk in the lemon juice, lemon extract and almond extract. Spoon into the prepared crust.

In a medium bowl, beat the egg whites and cream of tartar with an electric mixer on medium speed until foamy. Add the vanilla and the remaining 1 tablespoon sugar. Beat at high speed until stiff peaks form. Spread over the pie filling, making sure to leave no gaps where the meringue topping meets the crust.

Bake for 10 minutes, or until the meringue is golden brown. Chill for several hours before cutting.

Index

Underscored page references indicate Chef's Notes. **Boldface** references indicate photographs.

Conversion Chart

These equivalents have been slightly rounded to make measuring easier.

VOLUME MEASUREMENTS

U.S.	Imperial	Metric
¼ tsp	–	1.25 ml
½ tsp	–	2.5 ml
1 tsp	–	5 ml
1 Tbsp	–	15 ml
2 Tbsp (1 oz)	1 fl oz	30 ml
¼ cup (2 oz)	2 fl oz	60 ml
⅓ cup (3 oz)	3 fl oz	80 ml
½ cup (4 oz)	4 fl oz	120 ml
⅔ cup (5 oz)	5 fl oz	160 ml
¾ cup (6 oz)	6 fl oz	180 ml
1 cup (8 oz)	8 fl oz	240 ml

WEIGHT MEASUREMENTS

U.S.	Metric
1 oz	30 g
2 oz	60 g
4 oz (¼ lb)	115 g
5 oz (⅓ lb)	145 g
6 oz	170 g
7 oz	200 g
8 oz (½ lb)	230 g
10 oz	285 g
12 oz (¾ lb)	340 g
14 oz	400 g
16 oz (1 lb)	455 g
2.2 lb	1 kg

LENGTH MEASUREMENTS

U.S.	Metric
¼"	0.6 cm
½"	1.25 cm
1"	2.5 cm
2"	5 cm
4"	11 cm
6"	15 cm
8"	20 cm
10"	25 cm
12" (1')	30 cm

PAN SIZES

U.S.	Metric
8" cake pan	20 × 4-cm sandwich or cake tin
9" cake pan	23 × 3.5-cm sandwich or cake tin
11" × 7" baking pan	28 × 18-cm baking pan
13" × 9" baking pan	32.5 × 23-cm baking pan
2-qt rectangular baking dish	30 × 19-cm baking dish
15" × 10" baking pan	38 × 25.5-cm baking pan (Swiss roll tin)
9" pie plate	22 × 4 or 23 × 4-cm pie plate
7" or 8" springform pan	18 or 20-cm springform or loose-bottom cake tin
9" × 5" loaf pan	23 × 13-cm or 2-lb narrow loaf pan or pâté tin
1½-qt casserole	1.5-l casserole
2-qt casserole	2-l casserole

TEMPERATURES

Fahrenheit	Centigrade	Gas
140°	60°	–
160°	70°	–
180°	80°	–
225°	110°	–
250°	120°	½
300°	150°	2
325°	160°	3
350°	180°	4
375°	190°	5
400°	200°	6
450°	230°	8
500°	260°	–